NUTRITION AND KILLER DISEASES

NUTRITION AND KILLER DISEASES

The Effects of Dietary Factors on Fatal Chronic Diseases

Edited by

John Rose

Blackburn College of Technology and Design, Blackburn, England
Hon. Director, The Institution of Environmental Sciences,
London, England

np NOYES PUBLICATIONS
Park Ridge, New Jersey, U.S.A.

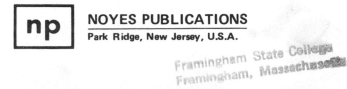

Library of Congress Catalog Card Number: 82-3401
ISBN: 0-8155-0902-2
Printed in the United States

Published in the United States of America by
Noyes Publications
Mill Road, Park Ridge, New Jersey 07656

10 9 8 7 6 5 4 3 2 1

Library of Congress Cataloging in Publication Data
Main entry under title:

Nutrition and killer diseases.

    Includes bibliographies and index.
    1. Nutritionally induced diseases. I. Rose,
John, 1917-   . [DNLM: 1. Disease -- Etiology.
2. Diet--Adverse effects. QT 235 N9758]
RC622.N885   616.07'1   82-3401
ISBN 0-8155-0902-2   AACR2

This book is dedicated to the memory of my brother, Isaac, a physician, whose work for his patients was cut short by cardiovascular disease.

Foreword

In this volume the term "killer diseases" is used to depict a number of chronic diseases leading to premature death. In our society, atherosclerosis and accompanying coronary heart disease, cancer and diabetes are among the most common. All of these diseases are of complex etiology and for this reason cause and effect has been impossible to prove. All of these diseases have a nutritional component either in their etiology or treatment. Since nutrition is one environmental variable which can be altered, the evidence for an association between certain nutritional patterns and these diseases is reviewed.

Presently, the association between total and saturated fat in the diet and atherosclerosis is a strong one. While most of the evidence is epidemiologic a limited number of experimental studies and a recent human intervention study support the view that high levels of dietary saturated fat and cholesterol will elevate serum cholesterol levels which, in turn, will increase the risk for coronary artery disease. Since the diet of many industrialized Western countries is high in total fat, high in saturated fat, and high in cholesterol, it would seem reasonable to recommend certain moderate changes to lower these components. This does not mean radical changes for most people but rather a change in emphasis away from fatty cuts of meat and dairy products without the fat removed, to leaner meats, fish, poultry, skimmed milk and skimmed milk products, vegetables and grains. As we shall see, such a shift in emphasis offers certain other advantages.

Cancer is a general term depicting the neoplastic growth of a variety of tissues. It may have many causes and, no doubt, different cancers have different causes. Two types of cancer, cancer of the colon and cancer of the breast, may be in part induced by diet. There are data from several epidemiologic studies that both of these cancers are associated with a high intake of total fat. In addition, cancer of the colon may be associated with a low intake of dietary fiber. The mechanisms by which fat and fiber may be involved in the pathogenesis of these two diseases is unknown, but it is speculated that in the case of breast cancer a high fat diet alters the female hormonal balance creating an environment more conducive to the growth of neoplastic tissue in the breast. In the case of cancer of the colon, the high fat diet selects a bacterial flora which metabolizes the fat in such a way as to release "precarcinogens." The low fiber diet results in a prolonged transit time for the intestinal contents and hence these precarcinogens have more time in contact with the bowel wall. Experimental studies are now in progress to test these theories. Whatever the reasons for the association, it would seem that a diet low in total fat and high in fiber may offer some protection against these two types of cancer.

While there is no evidence that any type of dietary pattern will increase the incidence of diabetes, there are numerous studies, demonstrating an association between obesity and maturity onset diabetes. In addition, weight reduction is the cornerstone of therapy in the obese diabetic. Treatment of diabetes should be aimed at reducing the incidence of vascular complications. To this end, a diet high in complex carbohydrates, low in fat and in saturated fat and low in cholesterol is indicated.

Thus for these three killer diseases a low fat, high carbohydrate diet appears to be useful. While the evidence that such a diet will affect all three of these diseases is not absolute, in my judgment it is strong enough to at least suggest that the general public move in that direction.

January 1982
Myron Winick, M.D.
New York, New York (U.S.A)

Contributors

Belinda Barnes
Godalming
Surrey, United Kingdom

Arnold E. Bender
Queen Elizabeth College
London, United Kingdom

Edwin L. Bierman
University of Washington
Seattle, Washington

Derek Bryce-Smith
University of Reading
Reading, United Kingdom

Denis P. Burkitt
Bussage, Stroud (Glds.)
United Kingdom

Alan Chait
University of Washington
Seattle, Washington

Ronald S. Goor
National Heart, Lung, and
  Blood Institute
National Institutes of Health
Bethesda, Maryland

Scott M. Grundy
Veterans Administration
  Medical Center
  and
University of California
San Diego, California

George V. James
Winterbourne, Avon
United Kingdom

Richard J. Jarrett
Guy's Hospital Medical School
London, United Kingdom

Carl C. Pfeiffer
Brain Bio Center
Princeton, New Jersey

Basil M. Rifkind
National Heart, Lung, and
  Blood Institute
National Institutes of Health
Bethesda, Maryland

Regina Schoental
Royal Veterinary College
University of London
London, United Kingdom

Dennis Shapcott
Centre Hospitalier Universitaire
Sherbrooke, Quebec, Canada

Hugh M. Sinclair
International Institute of
  Human Nutrition
Oxon, United Kingdom

Sir Thomas Symington
Troon
Ayrshire, United Kingdom

Richard W.D. Turner
University of Edinburgh
Edinburgh, United Kingdom

Gloria L. Vega
Veterans Administration
  Medical Center
    and
University of California
San Diego, California

Myron Winick
Columbia University
College of Physicians and
  Surgeons
New York, New York

Preface

Infective diseases are no longer a major cause of death in Western countries because of improved nutrition and reduced contact with pathogenic organisms. However, they have been replaced by a formidable array of afflictions which are now recognised to be characteristic of modern life in the West. There is ample evidence to support the thesis that inadequate nutrition is an important contributory factor to the alarming rise in prevalence of these killer diseases, viz. cardiovascular disease, cancer and diabetes.

This book [partly based on the proceedings of a National Conference on "Killer Diseases", held at the Royal Society of Medicine in London (UK) in May 1980, under the aegis of the Institution of Environmental Sciences] is concerned with a critical evaluation of the effects of dietary factors on "killer diseases". The scope of these considerations is broadened by analysing the effects of heavy metals and vitamin deficiencies with regard to birth defects and diseases of the middle age, the role played by some naturally occurring substances, including mycotoxins, in the aetiology of disorders in modern man, and the relation between trace substances and health. Particular attention is paid to the role of diet in all types of diabetes, and the importance of dietary management of this affliction is extensively described.

Other parts of the book are concerned with cardiovascular disease from a variety of points of view. Thus the evidence for and against the lipid and lipoprotein hypotheses is presented in detail, the point being made that other factors, apart from nutrition, may be implicated in the epidemic increase of the rate of "diseases of affluence". Another aspect considered in some detail is the relationship between cancer and nutrition and some conclusions are drawn about the mechanisms involved. Stress is laid on the ingestion of carcinogens with the diet and the role of endogenous carcinogens and co-carcinogens formed within the body. Particular attention is drawn to the role of pre-malignant lesions and also to repair enzymes.

The aim of this compendium is to review the present state of knowledge in a critical fashion without built-in prejudices and unsubstantiated theories, and

to possibly indicate future development. One has to remember that in developed
countries half of the deaths in middle age are now due to cardiovascular diseases,
while a quarter are due to cancer. Throughout the various papers contributed
by American and British experts there is a wealth of useful advice concerning
diet that may help to reduce the incidence and gravity of "killer diseases". After
all, in some populations (Hunza, Eskimo, some developing countries, Japan)
such diseases are either unknown or of low incidence. It is hoped that the sober
and critical appraisal of the current situation will be of some value in increasing
public knowledge and fighting the scourges of modern man.

J. Rose
Blackburn, England, January 1982

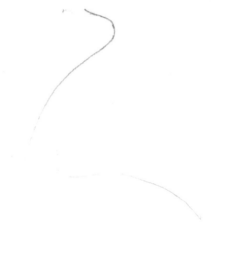

Contents

-1-

Diseases of Affluence

Denis P. Burkitt

SUMMARY

Infective diseases are no longer a major cause of death in Western countries. The main factors in their reduced prevalence has been adequate nutrition and reduced contact with pathogenic organisms. They have been replaced by a formidable list of diseases now recognised to be characteristic of modern western culture. Evidence is accumulating that changes in diet consisting primarily of a reduced intake of starch and fibre, and increased consumption of fat and sugar are important contributory factors to the rise in prevalences of these diseases.

REDUCTION IN INFECTIVE DISEASE

Prior to the last half century, the majority of deaths, even in Western countries, were the result of infective disease. This included many ailments that are rarely fatal in affluent societies today, such as tuberculosis, pneumonia, gastroenteritis, diphtheria, measles and many varieties of chronic sepsis. No longer are these diseases major medical hazards. McKeown[1] attributes the great reduction in the prevalence and mortality from these diseases that occurred progressively during the second half of the 19th century and the first quarter of the 20th century to factors entirely other than therapeutic medicine. He attributes improved nutrition, with resultant increased host resistance to infection, as the most important factor contributing to this improvement. The next most important was reduced contact with pathogenic organisms as a result of adequate sewerage disposal and provision of clean water and milk. Drugs played little part and only then after the discovery of sulphonamides and antibiotics.

The current major killer diseases in Western countries are non-infective rather than infective, with cardiovascular disease and cancer heading the list. As with infective disease, prevention is likely to prove vastly more successful than treatment in controlling this new epidemic.

1

Whereas inadequate nutrition was to a large extent to blame for high mortality rates from infective diseases in the past, it is faulty and often excessive nutrition that appears to be responsible for many of the diseases characteristic of modern western culture commonly and collectively referred to as 'Western diseases.'

WESTERN DISEASES RELATED TO DIET

These include such major maladies as coronary heart disease (CHD) now the commonest cause of death in affluent western societies; diverticular disease of the colon (DD) present, though usually symptomless, in about one-third of the population over the age of 60; large bowel cancer, the next commonest cause of cancer death after lung tumours related to smoking; gallstones, the commonest cause for abdominal surgery; appendicitis, varicose veins, obesity, diabetes, and hiatus hernia. All these diseases have been related to the diets which are characteristic of economically more developed countries. These have a low content of starch and fibre and a high content of fat and sugar. Hypertension is epidemiologically related to salt intake.

OTHER WESTERN DISEASES

No firm hypotheses have yet been formulated for other characteristically western diseases such as multiple sclerosis, Crohn's disease and ulcerative colitis. These diseases are universally rare, and in the case of some virtually nonexistent in rural communities in the third world.

There is no evidence that any of the above disorders was other than rare, or relatively rare, even in Western countries before the present century. Extrapolation from experience in other countries would suggest that the diets known to have been consumed in Britain and North America over a century ago would have been expected to be associated with relatively low prevalences of these diseases, all of which have today comparable prevalence in both black and white Americans. A generation ago they were much less common in American blacks and it can confidently be assumed that when their ancestors arrived in North America they cannot have been more prone to develop these diseases than are rural Africans today.

These diseases were uncommon in Japan before the second World War, but most of them have been steadily increasing in prevalence since 1950. In second and subsequent generations of Japanese emigrants to Hawaii and California the prevalences of these diseases are comparable to those in Caucasians. Although these diseases are rare in Polynesian island communities, prevalences rise steeply after emigration to New Zealand and adoption of a western way of life. In the case of some of these diseases, the Maori community are now at greater risk than are Caucasians.

These and many other similar examples indicate that environmental rather than genetic factors are primarily responsible for these diseases. The question remains as to what factors are implicated since the contrast in life style between third world and Western countries are multitudinous. Since all these diseases are related either directly or indirectly to the alimentary tract, it would seem logical to consider the possible implications of dietary changes before considering other environmental factors for which it is difficult to make hypotheses of causation that make biological sense. Only the diseases that have been specifically related to the depletion of fibre in the diet will be discussed here.

DIETARY CONTRAST BETWEEN POORER AND MORE AFFLUENT SOCIETIES

Although diets vary in types of food eaten according to climate and other conditions, there are certain patterns of nutrition that characterise communities with low or high prevalences of the diseases listed. In the former, some 70% of energy is provided by starchy carbohydrate foods retaining their natural complement of fibre. Fat provides only 10-15% of energy and protein, mostly of vegetable origin, about the same. In affluent societies on the other hand only a little over 40% of energy is derived from carbohydrate and approximately half of this is provided by sugar. Not only has cereal intake been considerably reduced, but most of it is provided by flour which has largely been depleted of its fibre. Fats, mainly of animal origin, account for over 40% of energy consumed and protein consumption is comparable to that in third world communities but is, as in the case of fat, mainly animal derived. Not only is the daily dietary fibre intake in third world communities approximately three times that of Western countries, over 60 g/d in contrast to about 20 g/d, but in the case of the former it is derived mainly from starchy staple foods and of the latter largely from fruits and vegetables. It is important to remember that high-fibre diets are also high in starch and low in both fat and sugar. The reverse is also true.[2] Although fibre will be considered in particular because of its neglect in nutrition studies in the past, it must be remembered that high fibre implies low fat and vice versa.

INFLUENCE OF FIBRE ON GASTRO-INTESTINAL CONTENT AND BEHAVIOR

Fibre in the diet influences every stage of food consumption and digestion. The removal of fibre from food reduces the necessity for chewing and thus increases the rate of energy intake.[3] The sense of satiety relative to energy consumed is reduced and this predisposes to over-nutrition with resultant obesity.

The energy from fibre-rich foods is absorbed from the bowel more slowly than that from fibre-depleted foods such as sugar. This reduced rate of energy absorption is protective against diabetes, high prevalences of which are related to consumption of fibre-depleted diets.[4,5] It is in the large bowel that fibre exerts its greatest influence and perhaps its major effect concerns the onward propulsion and final elimination of bowel content. The most important function of fibre in providing protection against certain gastro-intestinal diseases is its ability to increase the bulk and maintain the softness of colon content. Depending on the source of the fibre, this is achieved by holding water in the lumen of the gut or increasing the bacteria mass which constitutes the major portion of stool bulk.[6] The average daily stool output in third world countries is approximately three times that in Western countries, 300-500 g as compared to 80-120 g.[7] A deficiency of fibre, and of cereal fibre in particular in the diet is the major fundamental cause of the constipation which is so prevalent in Western countries. As well as increasing stool weight and shortening intestinal transit time, fibre alters faecal pH and influences the metabolism of both cholesterol and bile acids, mechanisms which have been implicated in the causation of both gall stones and CHD.

NATURE OF FIBRE

For long fibre has been misunderstood and wrongly considered to be almost synonymous with cellulose. The lack of satisfactory means of analysis was largely responsible for retaining, until recently, the misleading and meaningless term "crude fibre", routinely used in labelling food products and meaning only part of the cellulose and lignin in the diet. The most important components of fibre from the standpoint of function and disease are the non-cellulosic polysaccharides which were completely omitted by the tests for crude fibre.

SOME SPECIFIC DISEASES RELATED TO DIETARY FIBRE DEFICIENCY

1. Diseases Attributed in Part to Reduced Volume and Increased Viscosity of Large Bowel Content

(a) Pressures Generated Within the Gut:

(i) Diverticular Disease. The presence in the large bowel of a reduced volume of faeces, increased in viscosity, necessitates increased effort on the part of the muscles in the gut wall in order to propel intestinal content forwards. This raises pressures within the lumen of the colon and these are largely responsible for the forcing through the gut wall of protrusions of the linings membrane. These are the diverticula.[8]

(ii) Appendicitis. This disease is believed to be due to a somewhat similar mechanism. The obstruction of the lumen, probably due to the presence in it of firm faecal particles leads to raised pressures distal to the obstruction. These are considered to be responsible for impairing the blood supply, which paves the way for bacterial invasion and its consequences.[9]

(iii) Large Bowel Cancer. There are several current hypotheses as to the source of the carcinogens responsible for colo-rectal cancer. It is generally excepted that dietary factors are predominant, and excessive fat intake in particular. Whatever the causes of this disease, there is increasing agreement that fibre, and that from cereals in particular, is likely to be protective. Fibre increases bulk and thus dilutes carcinogens no matter what their cause. It reduces duration of their contact with the bowel mucose by increasing the speed of their onward movement through the gut. It binds various toxic substances rendering them innocuous. For these and other reasons it is believed to be protective against large bowel cancer.[10]

(iv) Haemorrhoids. The traditional concept of haemorrhoids as varicosities of anal veins analogous to the varicose veins in the legs or varicosities at the lower end of the oesophagus, appears to be no longer tenable. Hamish Thomson[11] has shown that three sub-mucosal vascular cushions surround the upper anal canal from birth and that haemorrhoids consist of a prolapse of these cushions after their attachment to the surrounding sphincter muscle has been ruptured. It seems likely that this can result from the shearing force caused by the passage of hard faecal masses through the anal canal. Thus fibre can be considered protective against the development of haemorrhoids. Other factors almost certainly operate in addition, but an increase in dietary fibre should in all cases be part of the treatment recommended.

(b) Pressures Generated Within the Abdominal Cavity: Not only does reduced faecal content and increased faecal viscosity lead to a raising of pressures within the gut, but it also raises pressures within the abdominal cavity during the straining of abdominal wall muscles necessitated to assist the evacuation of hard stools from the rectum. This is believed to play a role in the causation of at least two diseases.

(i) Hiatus Hernia. If a ball with a hole in its wall is filled with water and squeezed, the water is forced out through the hole. The abdominal cavity can be likened to such a ball, the hole representing the hiatus in the diaphragm through which the oesophagus passes to join the stomach. A hiatus hernia consists of the upper end of the stomach being forced upwards through the diaphragm into the thoracic cavity. During straining at stool, pressures generated below the diaphragm greatly exceed those above it, and it is not difficult to visualise how this may be a major factor contributing to the development of hiatus hernia.[12] Epidemiologically hiatus hernia has never been shown to be other than rare in communities customarily passing large soft stools.

(ii) Varicose Veins. All raised intra-abdominal pressures are readily transmitted to the great venus trunks at the back of the abdomen which receive blood from the leg veins. The blood in these vessels is forced retrogradely down the veins of the leg. In the less supported superficial veins this results in stretching of the walls above, and then at the level of, the first valve which when intact can withstand these pressures. When this dilatation separates the cusps of the first valve it becomes incompetent, allowing the retrograde flow of the blood through it. The pressures are then applied to the next valve lower down. Each valve becomes incompetent sequentially from above downwards and when the whole of the saphenous trunk is incompetent, intravenous pressures at the ankle can exceed arterial blood pressures. This is believed to be a major but not an early cause of varicose veins.[13]

2. Diseases Attributed to Excessive Intake and Rate of Absorption of Energy

(a) Obesity: Fibre in food provides bulk without energy, moreover it requires

chewing and thus prolongs the time spent eating. Foods rich in fibre have a low energy-satiety ratio, meaning that a sense of satiety is achieved before excessive energy is consumed and this mitigates against excessive energy consumption and thus protects against obesity. The reverse is the case with foods low in fibre content. Excessive energy then is consumed before satiety is achieved and this fosters the development of obesity.[3] Foods containing much energy but little or no fibre are sugars, fats, alcohol and to some extent white flour.

(b) Diabetes: Fibre in diet not only reduces the amount of energy consumed and the speed with which it is ingested, but it also increases the viscosity of the contents of the upper intestine and thus reduces the rate at which energy can be absorbed into the system. This in turn avoids excessive demands for insulin output and is considered a major factor protective against the development of diabetes. Contrary to the traditional practice, diets rich in carbohydrate, but with starch replacing sugar, and rich in fibre, are being increasingly used in the treatment of diabetes.[4,5]

SOURCES OF FIBRE

Not only do different plant foods contain different amounts of fibre but the proportion of the different components of fibre varies from plant to plant and also depends on the age of the plant. Different components of fibre exert different physiological effects. Just as vitamin B was considered a single entity when it was first discovered, but is now divided into a number of distinct vitamins, so it will happen with fibre. The all-inclusive term will be replaced by consideration of the cellulose, lignin, pentose, pectin, gums and other fractions. Largely because of their high water content, fruits and green vegetables have the lowest fibre content, never exceeding 3%. This is particularly true of plants like lettuce and celery which are often but fallaciously viewed as rich in fibre. Root vegetables collectively referred to as tubers and including, potatoes, parsnips and carrots have almost twice the fibre content relative to weight as have green vegetables and fruits. The fibre content in legumes or pulses, such as peas and beans is greater still but cereals are the richest source of fibre. Whole-meal bread contains about 8% but some breakfast cereals have much more fibre than this, the highest content being in All Bran 26%. Not only are unrefined cereals the richest source of fibre, but the fibre in them contains the highest proportion of pentose which is the component of fibre that has the greatest effect on faecal bulking and consequently on the diseases attributed in part to reduction in faecal volume.[14]

DIETARY CHANGES RECOMMENDED

It has been emphasised that high-fibre diets are also low-fat diets and vice versa, and that high-fibre low-fat diets are rich in starch and low in sugar. The overall dietary changes which could be recommended for Western countries as a whole would be in conformity with the goals of the McGovern Senate Committee in the U.S.A.[15] and would include:

. . . an increased consumption of starch foods, maintaining their natural complement of fibre and of cereals in particular and a reduction in consumption of fat and sugar. In more practical terms, much more bread but brown or preferably whole-meal to replace white; plenty of fibre rich breakfast cereals; less fat which implies less meat as even lean meat as presently produced is 40% fat; and a reduction in sugar consumption by about half.

REFERENCES

(1) T. McKeown, "The Determinants of Health" *Human Nature* 14-19 (April, 1978).

(2) H.C. Trowell, "Dietary Changes in Modern Times" in *Refined Carbohydrate Foods and Disease* (Eds. D.P. Burkitt and H.C. Trowell) (Academic Press, London–New York, 1975) pp. 47-56.

(4) G.B. Haber, K.W. Heaton, D. Murphy and L.F. Burrows, "Depletion and Disruption of Dietary Fibre. Effects on Satiety, Plasma Glucose and Serum Insulin" *Lancet* II, 679-682 (1977).

(4) J.W. Anderson, "Beneficial Effects of a High Carbohydrate, High Fibre Diet on Hyperglycemic Diabetic Men" *Am. J. Clin. Nutr.* 29, 895-899 (1976).

(5) D.J.A. Jenkins, T.M.S. Wolever, A.R. Leeds et al., "Dietary Fibres, Fibre Analogues and Glucose Tolerance: Importance of Viscosity" *Brit. Med. J.* 1, 1392-1394 (1978).

(6) A.M. Steven and J.H. Cummings, "Mechanism of Action of Dietary Fibre in the Human Colon" *Nature* 284, 283-284 (1980).

(7) D.P. Burkitt, A.R.P. Walker and N.S. Painter, "Effect of Dietary Fibre on Stools and Transit Times and Its Role in the Causation of Disease" *Lancet* II, 1408-1412 (1972).

(8) N.S. Painter, "Diverticular Disease of the Colon" (William Heinermann Medical Books, London, 1975).

(9) D.P. Burkitt, "Appendicitis" in *Refined Carbohydrate Foods and Disease* (eds. D.P. Burkitt and H.C. Trowell) (Academic Press, London, 1975) pp. 87-97.

(10) A.R.P. Walker and D.P. Burkitt, "Colonic Cancer–Hypotheses of Causation, Dietary Prophylaxis and Future Research" *Amer. J. Dig. Dis.* 21, 910-917 (1976).

(11) H. Thomson, "The Nature of Haemorrhoids" *Brit. J. Surg.* 62, 542-552 (1975).

(12) D.P. Burkitt, "Hiatus Hernia" in *Refined Carbohydrate Foods and Disease* (eds. D.P. Burkitt and H.C. Trowell) (Academic Press, London–New York, 1975) pp. 161-169.

(13) D.P. Burkitt, "Varicose Veins, Fact or Fantasy?" *Arch Surg.* 3, 1327-1332 (1976).

(14) D.A.T. Southgate, B. Bailey, E. Corinson and A.S. Walker, "Fibre, A Guide to Calculating Intakes of Dietary Fibre" *J. Hum. Nutr.* 30, 303-313 (1976).

(15) Dietary Goals for the United States–*Select Committee Report 96th Congress* (U.S. Printing Office, Washington, 1977).

2

Diet and Killer Diseases– Evidence or Opinion?

Arnold E. Bender

SUMMARY

The relation between diet and a range of diseases of Western society is still hypothetical. So many factors are implicated–the risk factors in coronary heart disease include unalterable factors such as heredity, age and sex, and abnormalities such as diabetes, obesity and hypertension–that environmental factors, of which diet is only one, are difficult to isolate. Almost every research paper gives rise to criticism and alternative explanations and so much conflicting advice has already been given to the public that the credibility of the medical scientist is low. Despite this lack of proof, which may never be forthcoming, it seems necessary to offer dietary advice to the public.

There is reasonable agreement that benefit is likely to result from a reduction in the consumption of fats, sugar and salt, and an increase in cereals, especially whole grain, fruits and vegetables.

It is not possible to state with any confidence that such modifications will postpone or reduce the incidence of disease but only that benefit is likely. Any stronger statements are certain to be refuted by others with resultant further reduction in credibility.

There has been intensive discussion over the past few years what public dietary advice should be offered, and indeed whether advice should be offered at all.

The problems are: (1) there is a sharp division between those wanting to advise the nation and those wanting to advise only individuals considered to be at medical risk; (2) it is far from clear just what advice should be offered (e.g., in relation to heart disease there are at least three different fat approaches–reduce total fat, reduce only saturated fat, increase polyunsaturated fatty acids); (3) it is far from clear which of the many dietary factors are to blame (again in relation to heart disease–fat, sugar, dietary fibre, etc.?); (4) the premise is that diseases of affluence have increased in parallel with dietary change but there is no agreement that the diet has changed; (5) the most problematical final point, which should be the starting point, is that we have no proof that diet is involved at all–the connection is hypothetical.

On that basis do we have the presumption to attempt to alter anyone's dietary habits?

The history of medical practice is littered with major mistakes. The litter may not be any deeper than that from other subjects but the results are usually far more dramatic. At the very least it behooves the modern practitioner to think very carefully before he repeats history.

It is not long since patients with myocardial infarction had to be rushed to intensive care units and receive very special treatment. In 1976 the Bristol study showed that patients treated at home did as well as those treated in hospital[1] and the Teeside Survey found a lower death rate in home treated cases[2] –a difference not explained by sending the more severe cases to hospital.

For years blood cholesterol levels were taken as the definitive index and high was bad; now we know a little more and look at high density lipoproteins where high is good. What is more sobering is the fact that many of these 'new' (1974) findings were made earlier (1951).

In the area of nutritional advice mistakes may not be drastic but it is already a case of crying wolf. Partly due to the writers of headlines, and partly due to the eagerness of some scientists to rush to the television studios whenever they have a (sensational) experimental finding, the public have been bombarded with 'facts'–so-called–about food until they are cynical, disbelieving or simply confused. Before we start another round of what some may call brainwashing, or nutritional guide lines, or controlling diets or simply offering unwanted advice–let us make sure that we are dealing with facts and not opinions.

EPIDEMIOLOGY

A great deal of the confusion arises from the misuse of epidemiological evidence–'everyone' says that this cannot be used to relate cause and effect and immediately uses his own epidemiological findings to do so. We continually read of the habits of the Masai, the Eskimoes, Indian railway workers and Trappist monks as if they provided causal evidence, and when they do not fit with the authors' pet theory supplementary theories are postulated. The low blood cholesterol of the Masai despite their high intake of saturated fat was attributed to genetic control but no evidence was provided for this suggestion. We even have the ludicrous report of a single human experience[3] offered as evidence.

For no clear reason there appears to be a desire to find a single cause of all diseases, starting with the evil eye, the 'vital' theory, the General Adaptation syndrome and proceeding to fat, sugar, salt, or lack of dietary fibre or vitamin C. 'Everyone' agrees that the diseases of affluence are complex and multifactorial, then proceeds to argue for a single cause–his own cause. More effort appears to be devoted to 'proving' one's case than finding the facts.

It is accepted that epidemiology provides only a starting point. The stages of investigations normally followed in attempting to find causes of disease, especially with vague links such as foods, are: (1) Epidemiological, (2) Retrospective studies, (3) Prospective studies, (4) Animal experimentation to investigate postulated mechanisms, (5) Short term human experiments to confirm postulates, (6) Intervention studies primary and secondary, designed to save life.

Most controversy rages around diet and CHD, and Ahrens[4] summarised the range of views currently held:

(1) The first group are those who conclude that the diet-heart question is utter nonsense.

(2) Advocates of low-fat low-cholesterol diets for the general public.

(3) Advocates of low-cholesterol, low-saturated fat, moderately high polyunsaturated fat diets.

(4) Sugar antagonists.

(5) Fibre advocates.

(6) A minority group that believes that the time is not yet ripe for drawing up national guide lines.

In this field it is as rare as it is in politics and economics to be brave enough to admit ignorance.

The practical problem is that with so many contradictory views any advice is certain to be followed by refutation by an equally authoritative group. It is probably true to state that every single paper reporting work on diet and CHD has been followed by an argument on methodology, statistics, or the results, or all three.

The unusually attractive theory that wine consumption is protective[6] was followed by criticism of the French death certification,[5] the subsequent removal of the questioned data,[6] and alternative hypothesis that it was really milk that is involved,[7] or garlic.[8] This is the way so many of the arguments seem to go to the impartial observer.

OPINIONS

The state of the art is well illustrated by the use of the term 'I believe' five times in one short article.[3]

The firmness with which unsubstantiated opinion can be expressed is illustrated by Yellowlees[9] with reference to the high incidence of peptic ulcer, CHD, hypertension and cancer that he encountered when he categorically stated 'the most likely explanation. . .was the kind of food that I had described.' He refers to the absence of fresh fruit and vegetables (complete absence?), the massive intake of refined carbohydrates (neither identified nor quantified), and the emotional description of white bread–'a white, inert, tasteless, constipating powder.'

Everyone appears to be confused. Minerva asked in the British Medical Journal (1979) 'Is the absence of any national food policy in Britain attributable to the lack of uniform specialist advice from the experts in nutrition and medicine as the Centre for Agricultural Strategy has recently suggested? Or has the impact of their advice been confused by the effective public relations campaigns by the food industries concerned?'

A small sample of statements illustrates the range of opinions on the subject:

> 'Only the optimists among us believe that obstructive atheroma in the coronary aerteries of our patients with angina might regress if we could persuade them to reduce the load of adverse factors in their life style.'[10]

> 'Authoritative statements on the causal role of high saturated fat, high cholesterol diets in the pathogenesis of atherosclerosis, based almost entirely on statistical evidence, are increasingly challenged.'[11]

> 'As evidence supporting the balance of probabilities in favour of a change in dietary lipid intake grows, epidemiologists are sustained or not sustained in their own hypotheses by the evidence of their own data.' 'Ex-cathedra statements based on undocumented debate in private sessions are no substitute for research data, epidemiological or otherwise, and must not be allowed to inhibit perfectly legitimate, sincere and well found initiatives aimed at altering the lipid component of the diet in the UK until definitive evidence supporting a contrary policy emerges.'[12]

> 'There is, as yet, insufficient evidence to justify a radical alteration in our present diet.' However the recommendation is 'Varied, balanced diet; aim at a modest reduction in fat intake; watch your weight.'[13]

A novel method of compiling evidence is by polling the workers. Many authors have quoted as support for their theories the poll conducted by Norum (1977) among 214 practitioners.[14]

Heart disease attracts most opinions but similar arguments rage about many other diet-related problems—breakfast and Crohn's disease; dietary fibre and 16 of the 17 diseases that have been correlated with fibre intake; sugar and diabetes; the causes of obesity; and the intake of salt, fat, protein related to cancer.

Sato[15] reported a decrease in the incidence of myopia in Japan of 50-70%, which he said is *most probably* a result of much improved nutrition (my italics).

Even apparently straightforward nutrition reports give rise to argument. When it was reported that extra milk did not affect growth rates of schoolchildren[16] and so implied that there was no useful function in supplying extra milk this was refuted because it is possible that it might have an effect on bone calcification (and so delay bone loss in postmenopause in days ahead). The author claimed that it was premature to conclude that free milk is unlikely to have any beneficial effects.[17]

Statistical methodology shares much of the blame for the confusion. All published results seem to be open to re-interpretation by employing different statistical methods and 'small differences that do not reach statistical significance' are freely quoted as valuable evidence.

The type of result is illustrated by an earlier finding of Ruffin and Cayer[18] who showed that of three similar groups each of 34 subjects, three complained of gastro-intestinal symptoms when given placebo, six when given liver, and nine when given yeast. Since, statistically, the nine is greater than the six, it was concluded that yeast causes gastro-intestinal symptoms.

This compares with some data on dietary fibre and diverticular disease.[19] Non-vegetarians without diverticular disease consumed *significantly* less vegetable fibre than those with the disorder (9.2±4.9 g compared with 10.7±4.2 g, i.e., 1.5 g less). In the same paragraph it is stated that vegetarians with diverticular disease appeared to have a lower intake of cereal and total fibre than those unaffected, but the difference did not reach statistical significance. On such flimsy figures opinion can masquerade as evidence.

NEED FOR MORE EVIDENCE

We are short of what appear to be simple facts. It is not even clear that dietary fat has increased in parallel with modern disease. One set of figures shows an increase from 98 to 130 g per head in UK since early this century; another set shows no change, namely 128 to 130 g. Mann[20] states that American intake of saturated fats and cholesterol has changed little or not at all since 1900 and the intake of polyunsaturated oils has doubled.

Recently the Butter Information Council published a fairly complete refutation of the evidence of the famous seven countries study of Ancel Keys on which the fat story is so firmly based.[21]

Evidence in most nutritional work is difficult to obtain. For example, even when it is clear that malnutrition is a major cause of death in developing countries it is difficult to demonstrate unequivocally the benefits of intervention. So many factors are involved–hygiene, medical services, education, vaccination, the economy, living conditions–and changing at the same time that the effects of food alone cannot easily be seen.

How much more difficult to select the food or foods which comprise only one group out of several groups of factors responsible, possibly, for our modern diseases.

The many factors involved in CHD can be grouped into three (Table 1)–those that we cannot change; those related to certain abnormalities; and it is only the third group, environmental factors, that we can, perhaps, change. Among these factors one sub-group is food and in this sub-group there are several different foods–each with its protagonist.

Table 1

A. Unalterable Risk Factors	B. Abnormalities That Increase Risk	C. Alterable Factors*
1. Sex	1. Hyperlipidaemias	1. Smoking
2. Heredity	2. Hypertension	2. Diet
3. Age	3. Diabetes	3. Water
4. Body build	4. Obesity	4. Exercise
5. Personality	5. Hyperuricaemias	5. Oral contraceptives
	6. ECG abnormalities	6. Occupation
		7. Emotional stress

*Cultural and environmental

DIETARY ADVICE

Many will agree that we do not have to wait for proof anyway, before offering advice, but this again will be a matter of opinion.

Before we consider what we might do it is necessary to enunciate the First Law of Nutrition–a complete diet adds up to 100%; and the Second Law–every dietary change has unknown repercussions.

The First Law draws attention to the often forgotten fact that any increase in a dietary constituent must be accompanied by a decrease in another constituent or constituents. It is often forgotten that treatment of diabetes with low or high carbohydrate diets (fashions change repeatedly) means that the prescribed diet is correspondingly high or low in something else–(and it would be more useful to state 'low' or 'high' in precise terms).

The Second Law emphasises the inter-relationship between nutrients–an increase in, for example, protein may require extra vitamin B_6 and magnesium; and increase in polyunsaturated fatty acids will increase the requirement for vitamin E. If these increased demands are not met then the dietary change will give rise to nutritional deficiency. Furthermore, nutrients react together and the effect of dietary fibre in rendering calcium, iron and zinc less available for absorption is a clear example. One would have to be wary of prescribing a sudden change to diet high in dietary fibre; and we certainly do not know the long-term effects of most of the changes that are talked about.

If we agree not to await the results of research before recommending changes then it is wise to recommend small changes at any one time with a correspondingly gradual effect. Do not eat anything in excess (an undefinable amount); a good diet should contain a little of everything, meaning a wide variety since we need to ingest a large number of nutrients.

WHAT ADVICE?

Shaper and Marr[22] in making strong, dogmatic recommendations for the 'postponement of CHD,' state that dietary recommendations to the public aimed at reducing the risk of CHD should not be confounded by other dietary recommendations which may be of general health value.

That implies that dietary advice will, rather than might, influence CHD. It makes the advice precise and dogmatic. If on the contrary, we do 'confound' other dietary recommendations, in other words we offer general nutritional advice, then we can generalise, and *suggest* that such changes *might* be of benefit and not pretend to offer virtual guarantees.

The dietary goals have been discussed many times and include reduction in fat (there is argument whether this should state total, saturated, specific fatty acids or even not reduce the fat but alter the ratio of P:S); increase in cereals with emphasis on whole grain, reduce sugar and salt, and increase fruits and vegetables, and avoid obesity.

Arguments can be put forward to suggest, but not more than suggest, that most people would *probably* benefit by changing their diets in this direction. It is not possible to be precise although it has been argued firmly that 'a reduction in saturated fat intakes and partial substitution by polyunsaturated fats–with the resulting change in the ratio of polyunsaturated to saturated fats–should be the basic dietary recommendations to the community.' (Shaper and Marr 1977.)[22]

On the other hand, it is equally firmly stated that 'the pursuit of these policies of fat reduction and more unsaturated fat is irresponsible, as it would have far-reaching economic, agricultrual and psychological effects. There might be quite unknown consequences of altering the nature of our dietetic fats. Even now we can be sure that a diet rich in polyunsaturated fats will increase the risk of gallstones.'[23]

The first McGovern Report (February, 1977) implicitly promised that adoption of the dietary changes would surely lead to reduced incidences of CHD, etc. The second Report[24] (December, 1977) stated more conservatively that such a change would decrease the probability of premature incidence of the disease (U.S. Government Printing Office 1977).[24]

It is the apparent precision and assumption of absolute knowledge that is wrong-headed in its approach and lacks credibility with the public. It is wrong-headed because we do not know that we can postpone CHD by any methods–that's my opinion, not fact. We can only state that if certain modifications are made in our diet then there will, on average, in general, be a likely improvement in health. (And not everyone will agree with that.) We cannot guarantee anything–hence lack of credibility. How do we answer the public when they relate stories of friends who have eaten fat, gotten fat, smoked, slothed in front of television and lived long and heartily while others who have obeyed all the dicta have died young? Do we tell them that the law of averages and the benefits of the next world support medical authority?

What we say and how we say it will influence how much notice is taken. It is extremely difficult to offer advice when it is not wanted and much more difficult to offer vague advice.

If we could only do it the best method is clear warning of immediate danger and evidence of immediate benefit. 'If you don't look out when you cross the road you will be killed' (yet people still do that every day). The worst method is vague generalisations–'it is believed that, on average, the risk factors might be reduced, etc.' but this is the nearest approach to truth (based on evidence not opinion) so this is what we have to say. Certainly if it is vague enough we will not be immediately refuted by others of equal eminence with the resultant confusion and disbelief by those we are trying to influence.

But is such vague and general advice really all that bad? We can still say to people there is evidence to *suggest* that they are eating more fat, more sugar, and more salt than is good for them. We can say that not all doctors agree on this (note that mere scientists' opinions carry little weight in such matters) but many do, so you would be well advised to try to improve your dietary habits since you have only one life to put at risk. You don't have to stop completely sugar and white bread and butter/margarine/cream or whatever, but rather modify your diet. Slimmers told that they must never eat chocolate again prefer to remain fat. Protagonists of wholemeal bread must learn that less than 1% of total bread sales are wholemeal–people do not like it. And even if many were persuaded that they must 'learn to like' wholemeal bread the amount of bread eaten by many people is probably too little to matter.

It is essential when trying to offer dietary advice to know the social customs and eating habits of those we are trying to influence. This was learned by the International Agencies many years ago but is still not understood in Western society. As recently as April 1980 at a discussion between dental health workers and nutritionists it was brought to light that dentists always told their patients never, never to eat between meals. Since so much of our social life is based on this very practice the advice was certain to be ignored. Another lesson comes from the same discussion. In the eagerness to stop people ingesting sugar between meals the dental health workers listed bad snacks (sugary) and good snacks–salted peanuts and salted crisps–at a time when other health workers were trying to reduce salt intake!

CONCLUSION

There is evidence to suggest that we do need to provide advice and that we can offer some advice. Public health cannot afford several conflicting advisers. We must bear in mind that any advice which is contradicted by subsequent knowledge will reduce credibility in the future. We must also bear in mind how the media sensationalise everything. The Royal College of Physicians used the term 'risk factor' for milk and this was modified to the headline 'the cow is a killer.' The advice must be reasonable, to stand a change of acceptance, must be explained, and any such campaign must last for a long time. Short messages such as news items are quickly forgotten. Above all we must be certain that the advice is worth having.

REFERENCES

(1) H.G. Mather, et al, *Brit. Med. J.* 1, 925 (1976).
(2) W.A. Colling, et al, *Brit. Med. J.* 2, 1169 (1976).
(3) H.M. Sinclair, *Lancet* I, 414 (1980).
(4) E.H. Ahrens, *Lancet* II, 1345 (1979).
(5) J. McMichael, *Lancet* I, 1186 (1979).
(6) S.S. St. Leger, et al, *Lancet* I, 1017, 1294 (1979).
(7) J.J. Segall, *Lancet* I, 1294 (1979).
(8) N.G.P. Slater, *Lancet* I, 1294 (1979).
(9) W.W. Yellowlees (1979). *J. Roy. College Gen. Pract.* 29, 7-21 (1979).
(10) *Brit. Med. J.,* Editorial ii, 418 (1977).
(11) *Lancet,* Editorial II, 337 (1977).
(12) V.M. Hawthorne, *Brit. Med. J.* ii, 186 (1977).
(13) *Family Doctor* (BMA Publications, London, 1979).
(14) K. Norum, *Tidsskriftfor den Norske Laegeforening* 97, 363 (1977).
(15) T. Sato, *Trans opthal. Soc. NZ.* 17, 109 (1965); quoted by D.S. McLaren, *Lancet* I, 655 (1979).
(16) I.A. Baker, et al, *Lancet* II, 575 (1978).
(17) F.B. Reed, *Lancet* II, 675 (1978).

(18) J.M. Ruffin and D. Cayer, *J. Amer. Med. Assoc.* 126, 923 (1944).

(19) J.S.S. Gear, et al, *Lancet* II, 675 (1979).

(20) G.V. Mann, *New Eng. J. Med.* 22, 644-649 (1977).

(21) M. Carruthers (undated), *Fats on Trial* (Butter Information Council, Kent, U.K.).

(22) A.G. Shaper and J.W. Marr, *Brit. Med. J.* 1, 867 (1977).

(23) J. McMichael, *European J. Cardiol.* 5/6, 447 (1977).

(24) Select Committee on Nutrition and Human Needs–U.S. Senate (U.S. Printing Office, February 1977, December 1977).

-3-

Nutrition and Cancer

Sir Thomas Symington

SUMMARY

It is argued that approximately 80% of human cancers have an environmental cause and carcinogens ingested with the diet or endogenous carcinogens and co-carcinogens formed within the body could be possible etiological factors. The carcinogenic nature of those dietary agents is based on animal studies and the problem of establishing an incriminating role for them in human cancer, is discussed. The activation and conjugation of chemical carcinogens, such as the polycyclic aromatic hydrocarbons, and nitrosamines, is considered and the role of the repair enzymes in protecting the organism is reviewed. Attention is drawn in man to some pre-malignant lesions as important sites for carcinogenic action and the relative risk of cancer developing subsequently in those sites.

It is only in recent years that attention has focused on the role of nutrition in cancer. Whereas the emaciated appearance of the cancer patient has been accepted as part of the disease, the systemic effects of tumours,[1] and the role of biologically active and non-active polypeptides formed by malignant tumours is now being studied, and their relationship with the physical appearance of the patient better understood.[2] The need to supply nutrients, by hyper-alimentation to the cancer patient, is under consideration in a few centres in the belief that this will allow the patient to withstand the adverse effects of the intensive radiotherapy and chemotherapy used in their treatment.[3,4]

This review will be limited to the possible role of nutrition in the etiology of cancer and will point to the difficulties and problems inherent in assigning a specific role to a nutritional cancer factor. This may be a dietary carcinogen ingested by the patient, either as a drug or as a normal dietary constituent which is metabolised in the body or altered by the bacterial flora of the gut to form a true ultimate or proximate carcinogen or a co-carcinogen.

A period of 10 to 15 years may elapse between exposure to a dietary carcinogen and the development of a clinically detectable tumour and during that in-

terval the patient may be exposed to a wide variety of environmental carcinogens (Table I) and co-carcinogens (Table II) in tobacco smoke, to irradiation,
and possibly to oncogenic viruses.

Table I: Known Carcinogenic Agents in (A) The Gas Phase and (B) The Particulate Phase of Tobacco Smoke*

Compounds	Amount in Smoke in One Cigarette, ng
A. Gas Phase	
Dimethylnitrosamine	5-180
Other dialkynitrosamines	2-80
Nitrosopyrrolidine	1-110
Nitrosopiperidine	0-9
Ayrdranine	24-43
Vinyl chloride	6-16
B.(1) Particulate Phase	
N-Nitrosonornicotine	140
Nitrosopiperidine	0-9
Nitrosopyrrolidine	0-110
Nickel compounds	0-600
Cadmium compounds	9-70
β-Naphthylamine	22
B.(2) Particulate Phase–Known Tumour Initiators	
Benzo[α]pyrene	10-50
Dibenz[a,h]anthracene	40
Benz[α]anthracene	40-70

*By passing tobacco smoked through a conventional Cambridge filter,
two separate phases are obtained: (1) Gas phase which is made up
of 90% of the whole volume of smoke but has fewer compounds, and
(2) Particulate phase which is collected on the filter as 'tar'.

Source: *Smoking and Health,* U.S. Surgeon General Report (1979)

Table II: Known Co-Carcinogens Present in the Particulate Phase of Tobacco Smoke and the Amount Present in One Cigarette*

Compound	Amount Present in One Cigarette, ng
Pyrene	50-200
Methylpyrene	30-300
Fluoranthene	100-260
Benzo[α]pyrene	30

*By passing tobacco smoked through a conventional Cambridge filter,
two separate phases are obtained: (1) Gas phase which is made up
of 90% of the whole volume of smoke but has fewer compounds, and
(2) Particulate phase which is collected on the filter as 'tar'.

Source: *Smoking and Health,* U.S. Surgeon General Report (1979)

At present, animal experiments are used to detect the carcinogenic effect of a substance. Whereas every agent known to be carcinogenic in man will produce tumours in animals, the reverse need not be true. Thus a dietary constituent or its metabolite which acts as a carcinogen or co-carcinogen in animals need not do so in man. This is the problem encountered when trying to assess the carcinogenic potential of the N-nitroso compounds.

In trying to understand the problem of nutrition and cancer etiology, much can be learned from past studies which established the carcinogenic nature of some well known chemical substances and their need of metabolic activation by the body before they could react with DNA or other macromolecules to produce their effect.

LESSONS FROM THE PAST

Early investigators did not suspect the existence, far less the nature or action, of potential carcinogens. It is not surprising that 140 years elapsed between the observation by Percival Potts that scrotal cancer occurred in chimney sweeps and the demonstration that skin cancer was produced in mice following the application of coal tar. Indeed there was a further lapse of 30 years before the concept of chemical carcinogenesis developed when Cook, Hiegar, Kennaway and Meynard reported to the Royal Society the induction of skin cancer in mice exposed to 1:2,5:6-dibenzanthracene which had been prepared from coal tar.

This important discovery stimulated research which led to the detection of numerous environmental carcinogenic hazards, and established animal testing of potential carcinogens as a vital step in drug safety evaluation.

The Role of Experimental Animals in Carcinogenesis

Animal experiments have established a clearer definition of a carcinogen as a substance which increases the risk to an animal of developing a particular cancer, compared with the risk when there is no exposure to the substance. Such a definition covers the development of spontaneous tumours but does not specify that the agent is the sole cause of the increased tumour incidence. Likewise it neither proves nor disproves that the agent acts synergistically with other endogenous or exogenous carcinogenic agents not that it is or isn't a co-carcinogen. Nevertheless, more controlled conditions can be established in animals than is possible in man, who is rarely if ever exposed to a single pure carcinogenic agent. Accordingly, much of our knowledge of agents as ultimate carcinogens or as co-carcinogens is based on animal experiments. Such agents are exemplified by some of the polycyclic aromatic hydrocarbons (PAH), aromatic amines, and N-nitroso compounds as well as some natural products like aflatoxin.

Animal Experiments and Co-Carcinogenesis

The classical animal experiments performed by Berenblum[6,7] laid the foundation for the concept of carcinogenesis. He showed that a co-carcinogen, croton oil, when acting alone will not produce skin tumours in mice. If, however, the animals receive a single subcarcinogenic dose of a carcinogen followed by repeated exposure to the co-carcinogen, a tumour will develop. Those experiments established solitary carcinogens as tumour initiators, a process considered irreversible, and co-carcinogens as tumour promoters, a state considered reversible.

Those early experiments laid the foundation for animal tests which in recent years have identified as co-carcinogens many chemicals of industrial and plant origin, those present in tobacco smoke as well as dietary metabolites such as the faecal bile acids.

Hecker and his colleagues[9] have identified the active principles of croton oil, as a series of phorbol 12,13-diesters which show varying degrees of activity as irritants and as co-carcinogens when exposed to mouse skin. Just as purification of solitary carcinogens allowed their interaction with DNA and other cellular macromolecules (RNA and protein) to be studied in detail, so purification and characterisation of the phorbol esters allows the use of more physiological concentrations of the co-carcinogen. In the strain of mice commonly used, tumour development can be achieved by an initiating dose of 0.1 μmole of 7,12-dimethylbenz[α]anthracene (DMBA) and a promoter dose of the co-carcinogen of 1 μg/mouse. Such low doses of initiators and promoters are well within the levels of carcinogenic and co-carcinogenic endogenous metabolites formed in the human body, and since activation of most chemical carcinogens is essential before they will cause mutation, this important process will be reviewed briefly.

METABOLIC ACTIVATION OF CHEMICAL CARCINOGENS

The somatic mutation theory of carcinogensis proposed in 1914 by Boveri[10] (1929) is still accepted by many. It requires that DNA should be the essential cellular receptor of the chemical carcinogen. If this were so, all carcinogens should be mutagens and positive mutagenicity tests would indicate potential carcinogens. When the simple microbial mutagenicity tests, available in 1960, were used, only a few known carcinogens were mutagenic, an observation which cast doubt on the validity of the somatic mutation theory of cancer. Since then, more sophisiticated mutagenicity tests have been developed. They consist of microbial and mammalian cell systems combined with prior *in vitro* or *in vivo* activation of the carcinogen[11]. Such tests indicate that most chemical carcinogens and many mutagens have to be activated in the body to form electrophilic derivatives which can react with DNA, RNA or cytoplasmic proteins.

Metabolic activation can be demonstrated for the potent carcinogenic polycyclic hydrocarbon–benzo[α]pyrene. This involves the heterogeneous enzyme systems present in the endoplasmic reticulum of cells from many animal tissues. They convert the highly insoluble, chemically inert polycyclic hydrocarbon into a soluble reactive ultimate carcinogen which is believed, but not proven, to be an epoxide or diol epoxide. The enzyme glutathione transferase, present in the cell sap, can conjugate the epoxide or diol epoxide and render it inactive. Thus, in assessing the ability of a cell to activate or inactivate a potential carcinogen, the balance of the two enzymes is important.

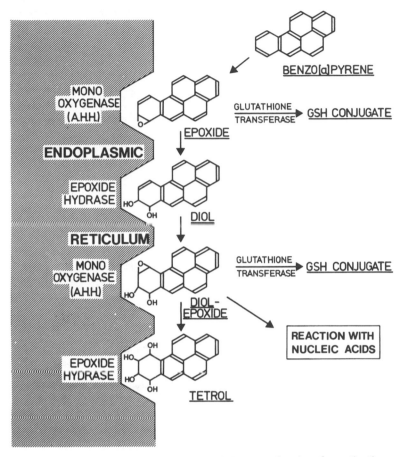

Figure 1. The cell metabolism of benzo[α]pyrene showing the activating enzymes in the endoplasmic reticulum and the inactivating enzymes (glutathione transferase) in the cell sap.

Although conjugation is an immediate and important defence mechanism for inactivating the potent polycyclic aromatic hydrocarbon, the soluble inactive form can now circulate in the body and be excreted or deconjugated by the β-glucuronidase enzymes formed by anaerobic bacteria which flourish in the human colon. The original carcinogen can now be reabsorbed from the gut, and if exposed to the many cells throughout the body which can reactivate it, become at that site a new carcinogenic hazard.

Much work has been done in recent years on metabolic activation of other carcinogens, and the reader is referred to the reviews on aromatic amines,[12] N-nitroso compounds[13] and on aflatoxin and other naturally occurring carcinogens.[14]

The N-nitroso compounds are, as will be seen later, important dietary metabolites and can exist as nitrosamines or nitrosamides. Both act as alkylating agents. The nitrosamides react directly with the target molecules, whereas the nitrosamines need metabolic activation before exercising their effect. The need for metabolic activation has resolved to some extent the remarkable species and organ specificity of the different N-nitroso compounds.

DNA Repair Mechanisms

While metabolic activation is necessary before most chemical carcinogens will bind co-valently to DNA, this interaction need not lead to cell transformation. A number of mechanisms exist in mammalian cells to repair any bulky constituents which form on the DNA. The helical distortion which results is recognised by an endonuclease which sucks and excises the lesion. This is degraded by the exonuclease, and a polymerase synthesized new DNA using the unaffected normal strand of DNA as a template. The ligase joins up the newly synthesised DNA to the original strand. This process is called *excision repair*.

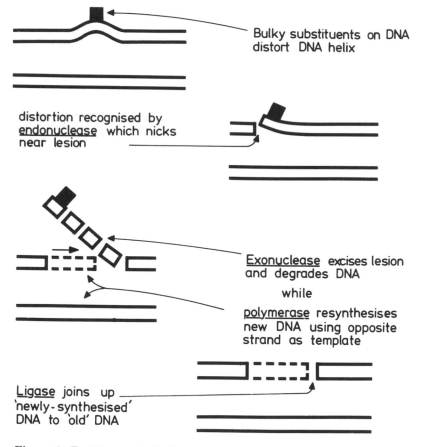

Figure 2. Excision repair. Bulky substituents caused by chemical carcinogens or by ultraviolet light distort the DNA. This distortion is recognised and the damage repaired as shown. From Roberts (1976) and reproduced with permission.

Alkylating agents, either carcinogens like the N-nitroso compounds, or certain cytotoxic drugs used in the treatment of cancer, as well as ionising radiation, can damage DNA. The effects produced vary from base pair substitution, single or double strand breaks, to inter or intrastrand cross-links. Those lesions are not always a block to DNA polymerase and the secondary damage caused to newly replicated DNA is amenable to a *post-replication* repair mechanism. However, in most instances the block to DNA synthesis caused by those agents leads to mitotic arrest, chromosomal damage and cell death. Reference should be made elsewhere for further information on DNA repair mechanisms.[15]

Chemical Carcinogens and Somatic Mutation

It will be clear from this short summary that most chemical carcinogens require activation before they bind co-valently to DNA. If the damage is not lethal, the repair enzymes and processes will recognise and deal with it. If cancer is a somatic mutation, the damage done by the carcinogen to DNA must be minimal and not recognised by, and therefore escape the effects of, repair enzyme. Such a minimal lesion could be a point mutation such as base pair substitution mutation caused by the N-nitroso compounds. Here the minor change in DNA is believed to result from the anomalous base pairing of 0-6 methyl guanine with thymine and not with cytosine as should happen. This base pair substitution will effect a change in only one amino-acid in the resulting gene product (Figure 3).

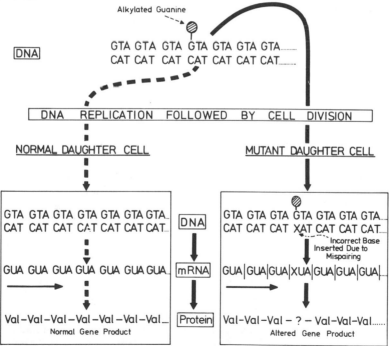

Figure 3. Illustrates base substitution mutation by aliphatic alkylating carcinogens like the alkylnitrosamines and nitrosamides. From Bartsch and Grover[8] (1976) and reproduced with permission.

NUTRITIONAL FACTORS AND CANCER

It is with the above background in mind that the carcinogenic effects of diet and nutrition can now be viewed.

Epidemiological Studies

Higginson[16] believes that environmental factors are responsible for about 80% of human cancers, and since diet is an important part of the environment, it is not surprising to find epidemiologists looking for a possible relationship between dietary factors and cancer. Studies have detected the presence of established carcinogens such as aflatoxin in the diet[14] and drawn attention to the role of dietary nitrate in carcinoma of stomach.[17] Epidemiological studies often begin by detecting an association between certain dietary components and human cancers and it is from such studies that more specific factors may emerge and their role as carcinogens or co-carcinogens determined by animal experiments.

Epidemiological studies first illustrated a relationship between dietary meat and fat and colorectal cancer. A series of studies showed the incidence of bowel cancer was associated with the concentration of faecal bile acids which was higher in the cancer patient than in normal controls.[18] Since animal tests indicate that bile acids are co-carcinogens it is tempting to ascribe an etiological role in colorectal cancer to the high faecal concentration of bile acids.[19]

Epidemiologists are now replacing physicians and industrial clinicians in drawing our attention to possible etiological agents in human cancer. At the same time, chemists, biologists and bacteriologists using animal studies have uncovered an important field of endogenous carcinogens and co-carcinogens, which are related to dietary metabolism. They will now be considered and for full details reference should be made to the excellent review by Hill.[19]

Endogenous Carcinogens

Intestinal anaerobic bacteria, by virtue of their enzyme activity, can convert many dietary products or their metabolites into substances which in animal test systems are shown to be carcinogens or co-carcinogens. While it is difficult to prove that such substances play a role in human cancer, their development and distribution in sufficient amounts in the body offer an explanation of the ubiquitous distribution of cancer and its development at different sites as the result of exposure to a single agent. This will be seen from the following discussions.

Products of Hydrolysis of Conjugates of PAH

It was shown earlier that PAH, ingested in the diet or inhaled in tobacco smoke, require activation before they will co-valently bind with DNA or other macromolecules. Likewise it is established that the liver can inactivate the carcinogen by converting it to a glucuronide, which is excreted in the bile. Some appears in the large bowel, where the original PAH is reformed from its glucuronide by interaction with the β-glucuronidase formed by the gut anaerobic bacteria. The PAH now formed must be reactivated by cells which contain the necessary heterogeneous enzyme systems, to become a potential carcinogen. This may occur in an organ quite remote from the original site of entry of the PAH. This explains why a carcinogen in tobacco smoke could be involved not only in lung cancer but in cancer of organs, such as bladder, which are quite remote from the site of entry of the PAH.

Amino Acid Metabolites

Tyrosine is metabolised by anaerobic bacteria to form the volatile derivates phenol, p-cresol and 4-ethylphenol which are co-carcinogens. They promote carcinogenesis in the mouse skin when applied locally to the animal which had received previously a single initiating dose of 7,12-dimethyl-benz[α]anthracene. The volatile derivatives are inactive as initiators of either carcinogenesis or mutagenesis.

Basic Amino Acid Metabolites. The formation by intestinal bacterial flora of cyclic secondary amines from lysine and ornithine is shown in Figure 4 and 500-1,000 μg of each amine is synthesised daily in the human colon and excreted in the urine. The cyclic secondary amines are nitrosatable substances and can be converted into carcinogenic N-nitroso compounds in the presence of a suitable nitrosating agent such as nitrite which is formed from dietary nitrate by bacterial reductase. About 100 gms of nitrate are present daily in the diet of the average European and American man, whereas the amount of dietary nitrite present is small. Both nitrate and nitrosatable agents can be found in saliva, gastric juice, vaginal fluid and urine and so the potential for forming N-nitroso compounds exists at those sites. However, most of our knowledge comes from studies of atrophic gastritis where the formation of N-nitroso compounds by the action of nitrite on a suitable nitrogen compound takes place at a neutral pH in the presence of bacteria.[19]

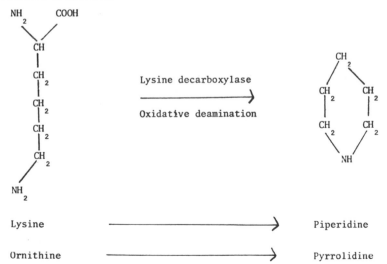

Figure 4. Production of the cyclic secondary amines piperidine and pyrrolidine. Modified from Hill (1980).

Information on the carcinogenic properties of N-nitroso compounds is based on animal experiments. Irrespective of its site of administration, diethylnitrosamine includes liver tumours in the rat, dibutylnitrosamine causes bladder tumours and dinitromorpholine lung tumours. Those observations either indicate that activation of the carcinogens occur in liver, bladder and lung respectively or the metabolite formed is particularly active at those sites.

Animal experiments have indicated in addition that the target organ for a particular N-nitroso compound may vary in animals of different species. Whereas N-nitrosopiperidine causes liver tumours in rats, it produces oesophageal cancer in hamsters. No conclusions can be drawn of likely targets for N-nitroso compounds which we have shown could be formed in man. In fact, while N-nitroso compounds are carcinogenic in all animal species studied, there is no hard evidence for their carcinogenicity in man. It is now established that, depending on the site, the time interval between the induction of a tumour and its clinical diagnosis, when it will weigh at least 1 gm and contain 10^9 cells, could be in the region of 10 to 15 years. The significance of this long delay can be appreciated when trying to assess the potential carcinogenic effect on stomach of a drug, like the H_2-receptor blocking drug cimetidine which is widely used in the treatment of peptic ulcer. Nitrosation of cimetidine occurs readily *in vitro* to give a nitrosoguanidine product, a specific type of nitrosamide which does not require activation but will begin to react and alkylate at its site for formation.[20] If nitrosocimetidine is formed in the stomach of patients with peptic ulcer from cimetidine and nitrite, it will begin to react immediately. Only small amounts of nitrosocimetidine will remain and be detectable in the stomach contents and disguise the fact that much has been formed and reacted. Brimblecombe, Duncan, Durant *et al*[21] found no increased risk of malignancy in a large-scale, long-term study in which cimetidine was administered to rats over a period of 24 months in doses equivalent to 60 times that used clinically. This is understandable since nitrosation of cimetidine in the presence of nitrite requires a low pH in the stomach, a condition not present in the animal stomach, but existing initially at least in the stomach of patients with peptic ulcer. "The key experiment which should define the carcinogenicity hazard associated with the use of cimetidine for maintenance therapy is the demonstration of methylation of the DNA in stomach epithelial cells after feeding the drug radio-labelled in the potential methylating group. The Radiochemical Centre at Amersham has now made available cimetidine which is tritium-labelled in the N-methyl group and the results of feeding experiments will appear in due course". (Professor A.B. Foster, Cancer Research London, personal communication.) In view of the clinical value of cimetidine, every effort should be made to assess its carcinogenic potential and not wait for 10 to 15 years to see if a gastric malignancy occurs. In the meantime, until the problem has been assessed, there is justification for supplementing cimetidine therapy with large doses of the nitrite inhibitor, vitamin C.

Bile Salt Metabolites. Deoxycolic and lithocolic acid are formed in large quantities in the colon in man, by the action of anaerobic bacteria. 200-600 mgs are lost daily in the faeces. Those bile acids have been shown to be co-carcinogenic in animals.

LESIONS IN MAN THAT PREDISPOSE TO CANCER DEVELOPMENT

It has been shown that carcinogens or co-carcinogens may be inhaled from the environment, ingested with the diet or produced endoginously by metabolic activity within the body and evidence for their carcinogenic activity is based essentially on animal experiments. Thus man appears to be exposed to endogenous and exogenous carcinogens which can be metabolised and circulated widely throughout the body. Repair mechanisms exist which can deal with severe damage done to the DNA by carcinogens, but in certain circumstances, where the damage is minimal, malignant transformation of the affected cell results. Animal experiments appear to indicate that the carcinogen is likely to achieve its maximum effect in tissues where the turnover of cells is greatest, where the carcinogen is activated and concentrated and more likely to gain access to cellular DNA or other macromolecules. There are a number of proliferative lesions in man that would allow the carcinogens to manifest such cellular actions. Those conditions are not in themselves pre-malignant but patients with them have a greater tendency to develop cancer than would be expected in the general public.

Women with atypical lobular hyperplasia of breast when followed up for a period of years have a four-fold relative risk of developing breast cancer.[22]

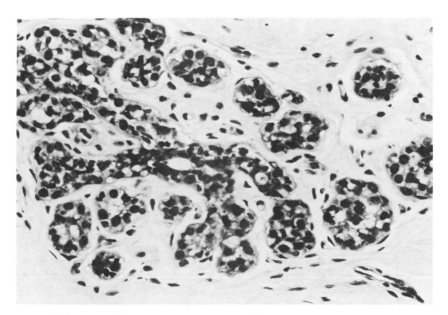

Figure 5. Atypical lobular hyperplasia of the breast and its role as a pre-malignant lesion.

Patients who develop atrophic gastritis (Figure 6) from a variety of causes have proliferating intestinal epithelium (intestinal metaplasia) in the stomach, as well as the conditions which predispose to the formation of N-nitroso compounds. Patients with ulcerative colitis develop polypoid lesions in the colon and have a high incidence of carcinoma of colon as do patients who harbour adenomatous polyps in the colon. Finally, the dysplasia of cervix, associated with sexual promiscuity, is a potential site for action by the N-nitroso compounds which could form there. If treated, the dysplasia is reversible and does not lead to carcinoma-in-situ or invasive cervical cancer.[5]

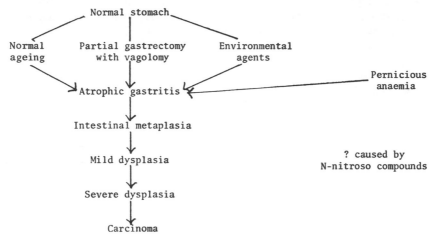

Figure 6. Postulated etiology of gastric cancer associated with high nitrate intake or with achlorhydria. Reproduced from Hill (1980) with permission.

Those are examples of four lesions which on their own are not premalignant but can under suitable conditions create the environment in which the multitude of carcinogens and co-carcinogens discussed could initiate and promote malignant transformation in cells. The identification and treatment of those and other similar lesions within the body is in my view an important step towards the elimination of cancer from those sites.

REFERENCES

(1) P.K. Bondy, "Systemic effects of neoplasia" in *Scientific Foundations of Oncology* (Ed. T. Symington and R.L. Carter) (Heineman, London, 1976) pp. 557-568.
(2) D.J.R. Lawrence and A.M. Neville, "Biological markers" in *Scientific Foundations of Oncology* (Ed. T. Symington and R.L. Carter) (Heineman, London, 1976) pp. 594-601.
(3) J.E. Rhoads, H.M. Rawnsley, H.M. Vars, R.W. Crichlow, R.W. Nelson, R.M. Spagna, S.J. Dudrick and J.E. Rhoads Jr., "The use of diuretics as an adjunct in parenteral hyperalimentation for surgical patients with prolonged disability of the gastrointestinal tract" *Bulletin of the International Society for Surgery* 24, 59-70 (1965).
(4) S.J. Dudrick, E.M. Copeland and J.M. Daly, "Nutrition and cancer" in *Cancer Assessment and Monitoring* Tenth Pfuzer International Symposium (Ed. T. Symington, A.E. Williams and J.G. McVie) (Churchill Livingston, Edinburgh, London, New York, 1980) pp. 357-372.

(5) N.A. Nealon and W.M. Christopherson "Cervix cancer precursors in young offspring of low-income families" *Obst. and Gyn.* 54 (2), 135-139 (1979).

(6) I. Berenblum, "The co-carcinogenic action of croton resin" *Canc. Res.* 1, 44-48 (1941).

(7) I. Berenblum, "The mechanism of carcinogensis. A study of significance of co-carcinogenic action in related phenomenon" *Can. Res.* 1, 807-814 (1941).

(8) H. Bartsch and P.L. Grover, "Chemical carcinogenesis and mutagenesis" in *Scientific Foundations of Oncology* (Ed. T. Symington and R.L. Carter) (Heineman, London, 1976) pp. 334-342.

(9) E. Hecker, "Some aspects of co-carcinogenesis" in *Scientific Foundations of Oncology* (Ed. T. Symington and R.L. Carter), (Heineman, London, 1976) pp. 310-318.

(10) T. Boveri, *The Origin of Malignant Tumours* (translated by M. Boveri) (Williams and Wilkins, Baltimore, 1929).

(11) B.J. Dean, "Short-term tests in the prediction of carcinogenicity" in *Scientific Foundations of Oncology* (Supplement) (Ed. T. Symington and R.L. Carter) (Heineman, London, 1980) pp. 37-48.

(12) D. Manson, "Some illustrative systems of chemical carcinogenesis *Aromatic amines*" in *Scientific Foundations of Oncology* (Ed. T. Symington and R.L. Carter) (Heineman, London, 1976) pp. 281-291.

(13) P.N. Magee, "Some illustrative systems of chemical carcinogenesis–nitrosamines" in *Scientific Foundation of Oncology* (Ed. T. Symington and R.L. Carter) (Heineman, London, 1976) pp. 292-301.

(14) G.P. Warwick, "Some illustrative systems of chemical carcinogenesis–aflatoxin and other naturally occurring carcinogens" in *Scientific Foundation of Oncology* (Ed. T. Symington and R.L. Carter) (Heineman, London, 1976) pp. 302-309.

(15) J.J. Roberts, "Some illustrative systems of chemical carcinogenesis–DNA repair and carcinogenesis" in *Scientific Foundation of Oncology* (Ed. T. Symington and R.L. Carter) (Heineman, London, 1976) pp. 319-333.

(16) J. Higginson, "The theoretical possibilities of cancer prevention in man" *Proc. Roy. Soc. Med.* 61, 723-730 (1968).

(17) P. Correa, W. Haenszel, C. Cuello, S. Tannenbaums and M. Archer "A model for gastric cancer epidemiology" *Lancet* II, 58-59 (1975).

(18) B.S. Reddy and E.L. Wynder, "Metabolic epidemiology of colon cancer. Fecal bile acids and neutral steroids in colon cancer patients and patients with adenomatous polyps" *Cancer* 39, 2533-2539 (1977).

(19) M.J. Hill, "Endogenous carcinogens in human cancer" in *Scientific Foundations of Oncology* (Supplement) (Ed. T. Symington and R.L. Carter) (Heineman, London, 1980) pp. 61-74.

(20) A.B. Foster, J. Jarman, D. Manson and H.R. Schulton, "Structure and reactivity of Nitrosocimetidine" *Cancer Lett.* 9, 47-52 (1980).

(21) R.W. Brimblecombe et al, *Gastroenterology J.* 74(2), 339-347 (1978).

(22) D.L. Page, R. Vander Zwaag, L.W. Rogers, L.T. Williams, W.E. Walker and W.H. Hartmann, "Relation between component parts of fibrocystic disease complex and breast cancer" *J. Nat. Cancer Inst.* 61, 1055 (1978).

-4-

Diet and Epidemic Coronary Heart Disease

Richard W.D. Turner

SUMMARY

Epidemic coronary heart disease (CHD) is due to changes which have come about in the way we live and primarily in the way we eat. Other risk factors, including smoking, hypertension, physical inactivity and stress may be additive in their harmful effects, but only food is a fundamental cause. It follows that the answer to the coronary problem lies basically in a more prudent diet. Ideally this should start in childhood, and preferably at birth or before with correct maternal nutrition during pregnancy as a preparation for breast feeding.

The characteristic features of our present unsatisfactory diet are that it is too rich in saturated fat, cholesterol, animal protein, refined food, dairy produce, fatty meat and meat products, hard margarines and cooking fats, egg yolk, white bread, sugar and 'rich' foods. There is too little wholemeal bread and other cereals, including the wholegrain breakfast varieties, pasta (spaghetti, macaroni, ravioli, lasagne), pizza, rice, pùlses, potatoes, greens, salads, other vegetables and fruit.

An inescapable fact is that vegetarians are not only just as healthy as others but, in some important ways healthier with a substantially lower incidence of heart attacks, strokes, intestinal disorders and some forms of cancer. In nutritional principle, a more prudent diet amounts to a return to a more vegetarian way of life which would be beneficial not only to health, but also to domestic expenditure, the U.K. economy, world ethics and animal rights.

Other risk factors for coronary heart disease do not appear to be important if the diet is a healthy one, but common sense dictates that no smoking, less alcohol, regular exercise and occasional blood pressure checks, say every five years, would be sensible advice.

INTRODUCTION

The motivation of a physician includes responsibility for patient care and for giving advice to patients and to their families who are at above average risk of developing the same disease, as well as to the general public, most of whom already have arterial disease although this does not necessarily mean they will develop symptoms. Many now seek advice and others would like to know without having to ask.

Usually it is the wife who asks, 'Doctor, did I feed him right?' and, 'What about the kids?' The first question is easy to answer because of course she must be reassured, but the second is intensely practical and should affect the whole family.

Further delay in preventive medicine is to condone an epidemic which is man-made and the answer to which lies in man's hands. As emphasised by the World Health Organisation (WHO), coronary heart disease threatens to become the greatest epidemic mankind has ever faced—unless action is taken. In other countries with a more realistic attitude, mortality from CHD has been falling dramatically for more than ten years, but not in the U.K. Most nutritionists lack the motivation of daily clinical experience and responsibility and many do not appreciate the strength of the evidence justifying action. Some demand 'more research' before action, but cannot define what research could possibly negate the necessity for a more prudent diet on the lines now widely agreed. Further research is only likely to indicate modification of detail. They find it difficult to accept that proof by dietary trials is unobtainable, but this conclusion was reached more than ten years ago.[1] It is the combination of clinical correlations, experimental work, epidemiology and laboratory research into mechanisms which provide confidence in advising a more prudent diet for the whole population and with the expectation of substantial benefit. There is no evidence to suggest that harm might result. In nutritional principle, the advice amounts to correction of radical changes which have come about and which were unplanned and untested for health.

Physicians believe it is not a matter of not knowing what to do or how best it could be done, but of motivating the many concerned, including the medical profession, the government, the Department of Health, the world of agriculture, food manufacturers, caterers and all concerned with health education. It is also of course essential to motivate the public. At present they are not well informed and there are many impediments to freedom of choice.

The doctor has in mind that sudden death is often the first, and often the last manifestation of CHD. Advice to individuals after symptoms have developed can obviously have little impact on an epidmeic. Doctors are not anxious to take action on incomplete evidence, but proof is unobtainable and the strength of circumstantial evidence justifies action. It is the purpose of this paper to explain some aspects of a problem of staggering proportions.

CHD has become the commonest cause of death in men after the age of 35 years. More than one-third of deaths occur before the age of retirement, and often long before, in the fifties, forties and even thirties. The fastest rate of increase is in the young middle-aged (35-44) years) group. Concern was being expressed as long ago as the 1930s, but the steep rise began in the 1950s. Now the incidence has flattened out, but at a high level, whereas in some other countries, including the U.S., Canada, Australia, Belgium and Finland, there has been a substantial fall over the last 12 years (Figures 1 through 4).

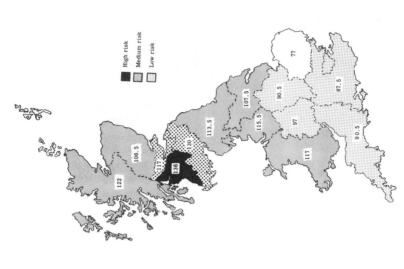

Figure 2. SMRs for ischaemic heart disease (ICD 410-414) in the regions of England, Wales and Scotland. Calculated using average number of deaths 1969-1973 and 1971 census populations. Males 45-64.

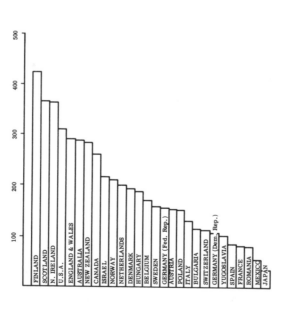

Figure 1. Mortality due to coronary heart disease: Males 45-54 yrs; Deaths per 100,000; WHO 1974-75.

MORTALITY
RATE
per 100,000

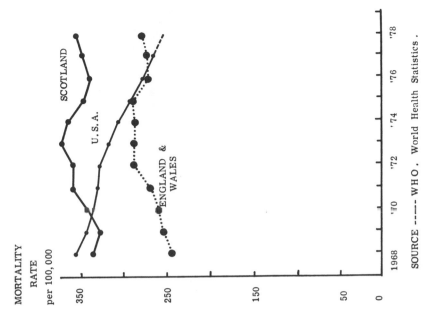

SOURCE ----- W H O . World Health Statistics .

Figure 4. Mortality rate for ischaemic heart disease.
Men aged 45-54: 1968-1978.

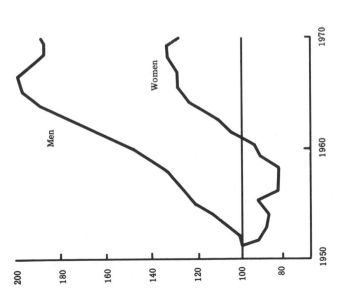

Figure 3. Percentage increase in death rates due to
coronary heart disease of men and women in England
and Wales in age group 35-44 years.

That the main causes of CHD *must* largely be environmental in origin and due to changes which have come about in the way we live is indicated by the steep rise in incidence in many countries; the wide population variations in incidence which cannot be explained by race, climate or geographical conditions; the experience of migrants from low to high incidence countries where they soon develop the same disease; and the changes in mortality which occurred in Europe during the two world wars. It is also indicated by the recent fall in incidence in a number of countries. It is estimated that improvement in acute coronary care has not made more than a small contribution.

There are only four behavioural changes to be considered:

(1) The food and drink we consume;

(2) The air we breathe (smoking);

(3) The exercise we fail to take; and

(4) The stress to which we are exposed or expose ourselves.

There is no evidence that smoking, physical inactivity, stress or diseases such as hypertension and diabetes are primary or essential factors, but abundant evidence that changes in our food structure and eating habits are fundamental and have invariably preceded the development of epidemic CHD. These changes have been well defined in population studies and the likelihood of causal relationships confirmed by experimental dietary studies in other primates and by clinical and pathological correlations together with laboratory work on mechanisms indicating harmful effects.

LESSONS FROM JAPAN

Comparative studies on the Japanese in their home environment and after migration to Honolulu or the Western United States are informative. The Japanese are a modern, industrialised, stressed, heavily-smoking and exceptionally hypertensive society. They are well nourished and have an attractive diet, but little CHD. This fact can be explained by their low (normal) blood cholesterol concentrations which can be correlated with their habitual diet. Characteristic features of this are an abundance of sea food in variety, but little meat or dairy produce, a high consumption of cereals (mainly rice), legumes and other vegetables, and little fat other than polyunsaturated soya bean oil.

In Japanese who migrated to the U.S. however and changed, amongst other things, their dietary habits, blood cholesterol levels started to rise and arterial disease developed. In due course, and especially in the second generation, they had developed much the same incidence of CHD as that in their host country. In those who stayed in Honolulu, the sequence of events was similar, but less marked, and they have an incidence of CHD which is higher than that in Japan, but lower than in the U.S. Only diet is likely to be responsible for these findings. In the cities of Japan the same sequence is now happening; the principal changes are increased consumption of meat, dairy produce, eggs and saturated fat.

The lessons seem clear. If the diet is a healthy one and *not* associated with a raised level of cholesterol in the blood, other risk factors, including genetic predisposition, are of little importance as regards CHD. Similar conclusions can be drawn from studies of other migrants, for example to Israel, from Italy to the United States, and in three populations of South Africa.

EPIDEMIOLOGY

The growth of epidemiology, the basic science of preventive medicine, is one of the most important medical advances of the century and has pointed the way to solving the problem of coronary heart disease. It is axiomatic that correlations, however strong, cannot themselves prove causality. However, given fulfilment of seven criteria they can be accepted, beyond reasonable doubt, as indicative of aetiological relationships.

The criteria are that the association should be strong, independent, graded, consistent, antecedent (definitely preceding and not following the onset of symptoms), predictive of future disease and, in addition, they should also be in conformity with demonstrable, plausible mechanisms and experimental evidence. It is difficult to believe that any scientist who studies the mass of evidence now available could doubt the fundamental relevance of epidemiology to the study of coronary heart disease. Up-to-date data will be found in the proceedings of a recent conference on The Health Effects of Blood Lipids: Optimal Distributions for Populations (1979).[2]

In the present context, the correlations of atherosclerosis and CHD with saturated fat, cholesterol, animal protein, hypercholesterolaemia, abnormal platelet function, smoking and hypertension have been supported by a mass of laboratory work on mechanisms and by experimental dietary studies. Correlations with sugar have not been supported by such studies.

There are many healthy well-nourished populations which do not have a significant problem from atherosclerosis and CHD even if they are heavily smoking, physically inactive, exposed to stress and have a similar incidence of diabetes and hypertension as that in countries with epidemic CHD. This favourable state is associated with the absence of hypercholesterolaemia and can be explained by habitual diet.

There is no reason to doubt that in the United Kingdom there could be achieved a similar favourable position if the problems of motivation could be solved. If children were healthily fed on the lines now widely agreed upon and good habits learned early were thereafter continued, the first step would have been taken. Wartime experience, in which 'rich' food was restricted, makes it clear that improvement in adults can come rapidly, presumably from reduction in the thrombogenic contribution to atherosclerosis and its complications. It is important to stress that smoking is not, as is sometimes claimed, the most important factor in CHD, but is only an important contributory factor if the diet is an unhealthy one. This of course is not for a moment to belittle the adverse dominant effects of smoking in relation to other diseases, including lung cancer, chronic bronchitis and emphysema. Perspective is important, particularly since persuasive advice on dietary correction is not always emphasised when encouraging smokers to abandon the habit. Coronary risk factors are not only individually adverse, but additive in their harmful effects.

Likewise in patients with hypertension, it is important not only to control the blood pressure, but to give advice on diet and smoking. In fact the risks of mild to moderate hypertension are almost entirely due to accelerated atherosclerosis only when the diet is an unhealthy one, as described in the present context.

Dairy Country Is Coronary Country

It is an epidemiological fact of observation and measurement that high consumption of dairy products is associated with a high incidence of CHD, and there is experimental evidence that the relationship is likely to be causal.

Finland has long had the highest consumption of dairy fat in the world, the highest concentrations of cholesterol in the world and the highest mortality from CHD.

In the Mediterranean and Adriatic countries, consumption of dairy produce is low because in general olive trees and pasture land are not found together. Likewise there is a low consumption of beef and little fattening of animals for the market.

It is noteworthy that the first cow to be killed for food in Japan was in 1931 and, although increasing in major cities, consumption of dairy produce and beef is still very low compared with Western countries. It is unlikely to be coincidence that blood cholesterol levels in Japan are now starting to rise, but there is also increasing use of hydrogenated fat by the food industry. The writing is on the wall.

In the U.K. consumption of dairy fat is high. It is not as high as in Finland, but that of fatty meat, meat products and beef fat is higher. In the U.K. more than half our beef comes from the dairy herd.

EXPERIMENTAL STUDIES

There are limits to direct observation in humans, but excellent experimental models have long been available, including in particular non-human primates. The most impressive studies are those carried out in the last 15 years in Chicago.[3-5] They have given ordinary Western food in comparable quantities, but suitably prepared, high in saturated fat and cholesterol, with a low polyunsaturated:saturated (P/S) fat ratio to non-human primates which closely resembled humans in their relevant anatomical, physiological and biological features. The response was a similar elevation of blood cholesterol and similar pathological changes in the coronary arteries followed by similar 'clinical' complications. In fact, the changes could not be distinguished under the microscope. Encouragingly, if the lesions are not too advanced, considerable regression may follow on changing back to their normal diet. Impressively, pathological changes do not occur or are mild and never obstructive if instead a prudent diet is given, similar to that now widely agreed for CHD prevention. It would seem to be stretching incredulity beyond reasonable bounds to deny the likely relevance of these observations to the human situation.

EVOLUTIONARY TRENDS

Evolving man branched from basically vegetarian stock. Later he became a hunter and gatherer of wild animal and vegetable life, but continued to live mainly on fruit, plant food and nuts for a million years or more. He was not bottle fed. Energy intake was matched by expenditure. His meat was lean and occasional, he had no dairy produce and there was no food industry. Eggs can only have been available from the nests of wild birds in season. Fat consumption must have been low and largely unsaturated.

A change began when he first started to settle as a farmer less than 10,000 years ago, domesticating a few animals and cultivating a few crops. Further changes were slow until about 200 years ago. Then, following the agricultural and industrial revolutions, there came a population explosion, movement to towns and the need for transportation and preservation of food. A food industry was born. It became possible to feed animals through the winter and then fatten them for the market. Later, meat was also imported. Margarine was first produced about 100 years ago. Only recently has there been a trend from poverty, which was the lot of the majority, to relative affluence, and with it a trend from vegetable to animal protein and an increase in the consumption of meat, dairy produce, eggs and saturated fat. Now most cereals, including flour used for bread, are refined, thereby removing the germ, the bran and many nutrients, few of which are put back.

Now, more than half our food is processed. The composition of fat, and the amounts of sugar, salt and other additives is unknown to the consumer.

Britain is not *well* fed. A sufficiency of what is considered by the Ministry of Agriculture, Fisheries & Food (MAFF) and the Department of Health & Social Security (DHSS) to be wholesome (safe) food is compatible with widespread *mal-* (bad, wrong) -nutrition. Clinicians know that an apparently healthy, well-nourished person may be dead within the hour from some complication of long-standing *mal-* (wrong) -nutrition which is the fundamental factor responsible for atherosclerosis as well as other diseases.

Our present diet is uniquely abnormal. Malnutrition from undernutrition and deficiency disease has been replaced by that from overnutrition and imbalance of nutrients, notably the fatty acids. The new era of 'convenience' and 'fast' foods is a mixed blessing and a matter of major nutritional concern.

THE PRUDENT DIET

Over the past twelve years numerous working parties from many different countries concerned about epidemic CHD have reviewed the relevant research on likely causal factors (Table I). Over such a long period the evidence was by no means always the same as new work was published, but there was of course overlap as regards key studies, especially those on epidemiology and experimental work. The working parties were entirely independent of each other and of vested interests, and were appointed by an appropriate authority. Understandably, each was mainly concerned with the problems of their own country, but took full account of similar epidemics occurring in other populations. No comparable matter can have been subjected to more rigorous examination or research, and remarkably similar recommendations were made by each working party. No conflicting evidence that stands up to critical examination was found and no contrary report of a similar nature has been published.

Table I: Recommendations of 20 Committees on Food and Coronary Heart Disease

	General Population (GP) High Risk Group (HR)	Fat Content of Total Energy (%)	Increased PUFA	PUFA-SAFA Ratio	Daily Dietary Cholesterol (mg)	Reduction of Sugar	Labelling of Fat Content of Foods
Norway, Sweden and Finland 1968[1]	GP	25–35	Yes	–	–	Yes	Yes
United States 1970 Inter-Society[2]	GP HR	<35	Yes	1.0	<300	–	Yes
New Zealand 1971 Heart Foundation[3]	GP	35	–	–	300–600	–	Yes
	HR	35	Yes	1.0	300–600	–	Yes
New Zealand 1971 Royal Society[4]	GP	–	No	–	Reduce	–	–
	HR	Avoid excess saturated fat	Yes	–	Reduce	–	–
United States 1972 American Health Foundation[5]	GP	35	Yes	1.0	300	Yes	Yes
United States 1972 American Medical Association[6]	HR	*	Yes	–	Reduce	–	Yes
International Society of Cardiology 1973[7]	HR	<30	Yes	>1.0	<300	–	Yes
United States 1973 American Heart Association[8]	GP	35	Yes	1.0	300	Yes	Yes
The Netherlands 1973[9]	GP	35	Yes	1.0	250–300	Yes	Yes
United States 1973 White House Conference[10]	GP	35	Yes	–	300	–	Yes
Australia 1974 National Heart Foundation[11]	GP HR	30–35	Yes	1.5	<300	– Yes	–
United Kingdom 1974 DHSS (COMA)[12]	GP	**	No	–	–	Yes	–
Germany 1975 (Federal Republic)[13]	GP	Reduce saturated fat	Yes	–	300	–	–
Australia 1975 Academy of Science[14]	GP	35	Yes	1.0	<350	Yes	Yes
United Kingdom 1976 Royal College of Physicians and British Cardiac Society[15]	GP	Towards 35	Yes	–	Reduce	Yes	Yes
Norway 1975–76 Ministry of Agriculture[16]	GP	35	Yes	0.5	Doctor's de-	Yes	Yes
	HR	35	Yes	1.0	cision	Yes	Yes
Canada 1976 Health & Welfare[17]	GP	30–35	Yes	–	400	Yes	Yes
	HR	30–35	Yes	–	400	Yes	Yes
United States 1977 Senate Committee[18]	GP	30	Yes	1.0	300	Yes	–
	HR	30	Yes	1.0	300	Yes	–
FAO-WHO 1978[19]	GP	30–35	Yes	1.0	<300	–	–
European Society of Cardiology 1978[20]	HR	30	Yes	1.0	<300	Yes	–

Note: DHSS (COMA) is the Department of Health & Social Security (Committee on Medical Aspects); and FAO-WHO is the Food & Agriculture Organisation (United Nations) and World Health Organisation.

*Substantial decrease in saturated fat.

**Reduce total fat, especially saturated.

(continued)

Table I: continued

(1) Official collective recommendation on diet in the Scandinavian countries, *Nutr. Revs.* 26, 259 (1968).
(2) Inter-Society Commission for Heart Disease Resources, "Primary prevention of atherosclerotic disease, *Circ.* 42, A55 (1970).
(3) National Heart Foundation of New Zealand, "Coronary heart disease." P.O. Box 17128, Green Lane, Auckland 5 (1971).
(4) Royal Society of New Zealand, "Coronary heart disease." P.O. Box 12249, Wellington (1971).
(5) American Health Foundation, "Position statement on diet and coronary heart disease," *Prev. Med.* 1, 255 (1972).
(6) American Medical Association, "Diet and coronary heart disease," *Nutr. Revs.* 30, 223 (1972).
(7) International Society of Cardiology, "Myocardial infarction. How to prevent. How to rehabilitate" (1070).
(8) American Heart Association, "Diet and coronary heart disease" (44 East 23rd Street, New York, N.Y. 10010, 1973).
(9) Netherlands Nutritional Council, "Recommendations on amount and nature of dietary fats," *Voeding* 34, 552 (1973).
(10) White House Conference, USA, "Atherosclerotic disease, diabetes and hypertension: background considerations," *US Nutrition Policies in the Seventies* (1973) chapter 4.
(11) National Heart Foundation of Australia, "Dietary fat and coronary heart disease," *Med. J. Austral.* 1, 575, 616, 663 (1974).
(12) Department of Health & Social Security (COMA), "Diet and coronary heart disease" (HMSO, London, 1974).
(13) Editorial, "Dietary fat and degenerative vascular diseases," *Nutr. Metab.* 18, 113 (German Federal Republic, 1975).
(14) Australian Academy of Science, "Diet and coronary heart disease," *Report* No. 18 (1975).
(15) Royal College of Physicians of London and British Cardiac Society, "Prevention of coronary heart disease," *J. Roy. Coll. Phys. Lond.* 10, 213 (1976).
(16) Royal Norwegian Ministry of Agriculture–Report No. 32 to the Storting, "Norwegian nutrition and food policy." (National Nutritional Council, Box 8139, Oslo 1, 1975-1976).
(17) Report to the Minister of National Health & Welfare, "Diet and cardiovascular disease" (Health & Welfare, Canada, 1976).
(28) U.S. Senate Committee on Nutrition and Human Needs, "Dietary goals for the United States" (Washington, DC, 1977).
(19) FAO-WHO Expert Consultation, "Dietary fats and oils in human consumption" (Rome, 1977).
(20) European Society of Cardiology, *Preventing Coronary Heart Disease* (Pub. van Gorcum, Assen, The Netherlands, 1978).

The answer to the coronary problem lies in dietary correction or, in nutritional principle, to 'changing back'. The so-called 'prudent' diet, now widely agreed to, has been well researched and is soundly based. The justification for change is to be found in the reports of the working parties and in the research papers they used as evidence, together with up-to-date reviews and the Proceedings of the Conference referred to above.[2]

Table II: Twelve Dietary Goals

(1) Match energy intake by expenditure.

(2) Decrease consumption of saturated fat.

(3) Partially replace saturated fat by polyunsaturated fat at table and in cooking.

(4) Decrease consumption of cholesterol.

(5) Decrease consumption of animal protein, except fish.

(6) Increase consumption of protein from mixed vegetable sources.

(7) Decrease consumption of white bread and other refined cereals.

(8) Increase consumption of wholemeal bread and other unrefined cereals.

(9) Increase consumption of potatoes, salads, other vegetables, fruits and nuts.

(10) Increase consumption of fibre.

(11) Decrease consumption of sugar.

(12) Decrease consumption of salt.

Notes on the Above

(1) In particular, decrease excess of 'empty' calories from sugar and alcohol as well as saturated fat.

(2) This includes dairy fat, meat fat and food industry fat in the form of hard margarines, cooking fat and 'rich food'.

(3) These include the polyunsaturated margarines and oils together with fish and green leafy vegetables.

(4) This includes meat, dairy produce and egg yolk.

(5) This includes meat and milk.

(6) This includes bread and other cereals, pulses (beans, peas, lentils) and potatoes.

(7) and (8) This will improve consumption of fibre and many other nutrients.

(9) This group includes minerals, vitamins and fibre.

(10) Fibre is a constituent of all plant food, but there is none in that of animal origin. Cereals, vegetables and fruit provide different types of fibre.

(11) This includes not only sugar added at table and in cooking, but most soft drinks and confectionery.

(12) This includes not only salt added at table and in cooking, but salty foods and salt added to many products by the food industry.

Groups 2, 4 and 5 are interrelated, as are groups 3, 6-10.

WHAT TO EAT

In summary and 'in general' (which indicates no prohibitions):

Avoid top of milk and cream. Eat butter sparingly. Instead, use a polyunsaturated margarine;

Avoid all hard margarines, cooking fats and shortening sold in packets. Instead use a polyunsaturated oil or margarine;

Eat less meat, choose only lean meat and remove visible fat. Restrict fatty meat products, such as mince, sausages, hamburgers, pies, corned beef and other sliced meats. Use meat more as a flavouring agent than main constituent of a meal. Avoid cooking in animal fats;

Instead of meat, choose more fish and poultry. Have less protein from animal sources and more from mixed vegetable sources, which include cereals, pulses and potatoes;

Cheese dishes make a useful alternative to meat;

Have more cereals as wholemeal bread, including sandwiches and snacks on toast; wholegrain crispbreads; flour, including pasta (spaghetti, macaroni, ravioli, canneloni, lasagne, etc.) and pizza; breakfast cereals, including porridge, muesli and whole grain varieties, such as shredded wheat; rice; oatmeal and barley to thicken soups and stews;

Have more vegetables, including potatoes, preferably baked or boiled in their skins; salads; greens; pulses (beans, peas, lentils); onions; fruit and nuts;

Restrict egg yolk to not more than three each week.

A return to a much more vegetarian and much healthier diet is implicit in these recommendations.

The dietary goals can be translated into simple recommendations about choosing the right foods. The advice is straightforward and easy to accept. Fortunately it is more economical. There can be great variety, as can be seen from the numerous recipe books available.

THREE IMPORTANT DIETARY SWITCHES

The dietary recommendations include three important 'switches' or substitutions.

Fat

A fat switch to polyunsaturated margarines and oils is an essential component of a more prudent diet in a country with a high incidence of atherosclerosis, heart attacks and stroke.

Consequently, caterers should be encouraged to offer a choice and to declare what fat/oil is being used for cooking.

A subsidised polyunsaturated cooking oil could be a profitable health investment for the government if used by caterers, the food industry and in the home. Phasing out of hydrogenated (and thereby saturated) oils and imported, saturated tropical oils, such as coconut, palm and palm kernel, which are widely used by the food industry is highly desirable.

Protein

A partial (or, if desired, complete) protein switch to mixed vegetable sources would reduce consumption of saturated fat and cholesterol and increase that of fibre in variety.

Carbohydrate

A carbohydrate switch away from sugar and white bread to wholemeal bread, other cereals and potatoes would be much more nutritious.

EMPTY CALORIES

Sugar, saturated fat and alcohol are three sources of 'empty' calories which have little or no nutritional value, but contribute to obesity.

There is a high concentration of sugar in most soft drinks and sugar is added by the food industry to a huge range of products.

MEAT, DAIRY PRODUCE AND EGGS IN PERSPECTIVE

Meat, dairy produce and eggs can provide important nutrients, but are not *essential* body-building protective foods, as still sometimes taught. Rather they should be considered as luxuries many enjoy and for which most are prepared to pay, but are nutritionally superfluous.

On the contrary, when consumed in present-day excess these three common components of the diet constitute, beyond reasonable doubt, the principal dietary risk factors for epidemic CHD. They provide on average 75% of the saturated fat and 90% of the cholesterol in the diet.

Meat

It has long been standard textbook teaching that meat is unnecessary for good health at any age. It does not, as commonly supposed, increase strength or virility. Meat does supply first class protein, by which is meant all the essential amino acids. However, to the clinician it is not the *best* source owing to the associated saturated fat and cholesterol. Protein from mixed vegetable sources does not have these disadvantages. It also provides all the essential amino acids, but *without* saturated fat and cholesterol, and *with* fibre in variety. At present a huge excess of carcass fat goes into meat products or is used for cooking by caterers and in the home.

It is important for children to learn that the sole merits of meat are sensory and therefore a matter of personal choice, and not health. Vegetarians are not only just as healthy as others, but in some important ways substantially healthier. They have a lower incidence of obesity, heart attacks, strokes and a variety of intestinal disorders, and some forms of cancer, including that of the breast and colon.

Meat is also relatively expensive. Present-day high consumption amounts, on average, to about one-third of the family food budget. Its production is also helping to ruin the U.K. economy owing to the high cost of important animal feed and of factory farming. In addition, there is also a rapidly increasing problem of world ethics with the population of undernourished developing countries expected to double within about 30 years. It will become increasingly difficult to justify feeding so much by way of cereals and protein concentrates to animals when they could be consumed directly by humans.

Milk

Milk is the major product of our farms, but its value as a food has been exaggerated. It is necessary to be objective. The reputation of milk was gained in the days of widespread undernutrition and deficiency disease. In 1934 school milk was provided primarily to benefit the producers owing to the surplus production which existed at that time. Under-privileged children benefited from the nutrients in the skim. It was not at that time appreciated that arterial damage might result from the fat when consumed in excess. Milk is a customary, convenient and versatile component of the U.K. diet but, with 20% of the EEC population, we consume more than 40% of the milk, and it is the richest in cream except for Ireland. There is no nutritional sense in this.

A similar situation now as regards butter has recently arisen in the EEC. We have the paradox that the DHSS has said, in effect, eat less butter on health grounds, but the subsidy from MAFF is to reduce the price and thereby encourage consumption on political grounds. This is but one example of the need for co-ordination by governments.

One goal of a more prudent diet could be to halve the fat content of standard milk below the present average of 3.8%. The difference would not be noticed. Likewise, the ready availability of lower fat milks and milk products, including cheeses, as in other EEC countries, would be welcome. The Hannah Dairy Research Institute has the necessary knowledge and expertise to market such products, but has been inhibited by the Milk Marketing Board against the interests of the consumers.

Children who dislike milk, or are allergic to it, need never be persuaded, and extra full-cream milk is undesirable on health grounds. In Sweden children have been given only skimmed milk for many years, and now find other milk 'too rich' for their taste.

Butter

As a component of the U.K. diet, butter has little or no nutritional value. It provides only calories and two vitamins (A and D), which are not in short supply. On the other hand, it is very rich in saturated fat and cholesterol, but very low in essential polyunsaturated fatty acids. When added to the daily feed of many species, butter, like other saturated fat, raises the level of cholesterol in the blood and produces pathological changes in the arteries similar to atherosclerosis in humans.

Adults are free to choose, but it is better for children not to acquire the taste for butter. Most have no preference and find the soft margarines easier to spread. Just as they should learn to 'pour off the top', they should also be told that, 'butter isn't good for you'.

On the other hand, since the pleasant flavour of butter is due to butyric acid, there is scope for enterprise by the margarine manufacturers and, meanwhile, for 'butter-mixes' with polyunsaturated margarine to be encouraged.

Since we import 70% of our butter (and 40% of the cheese), it would seem desirable for this to be phased out and for the U.K. to become self-sufficient.

The Centre for Agricultural Strategy at the University of Reading has suggested how the dairy industry could adapt to such a change in consumption to mutual advantage, but in 1979 no less than £12 million was spent by the Milk Marketing Boards on promoting full-fat dairy produce despite the recommendations of the DHSS and of the Joint Working Party of the Royal College of Physicians and British Cardiac Society. It also seems reasonable to suggest that there should be limits to promotion, as with the tobacco industry. It is paradoxical, to say the least, that the Ministry of Agriculture should subsidise butter in order to reduce the price and increase consumption, and thereby reduce the size of the 'butter mountain' to which we have to contribute.

Eggs

Eggs are nutritious, but their contribution to recommended nutrient requirements is, in the average diet, small. The problem with eggs is the very high concentration of cholesterol in the yolk. It can be calculated that without drastic reduction of meat and dairy produce, which few would want to accept, restriction of egg yolk to not more than three per week is necessary to reach the 'goal'. On the other hand, the white of egg is useful in cooking and is not of dietary concern as regards CHD.

If it were true *primary* prevention against the development of atherosclerosis which most of the population required, and if the partial fat and protein switches were accepted, then, as discussed later, there would be relatively little concern about eggs. The importance of dietary cholesterol depends upon the fat content and fatty acid composition of the diet. However, in the U.K. most adults and many children already have atherosclerosis and what is required in effect is *secondary* prevention aimed at its arrest and regression, and the prevention of thrombo-embolic complications. This is a very different situation. The relevance of dietary imprudence is the high risk of being the victim of an epidemic in 'the prime of life'.

Tertiary prevention is the appropriate term for those who have already developed symptoms.

Margarines and Cooking Fats

All margarines and cooking fats sold in packets are, like butter, hydrogenated and thereby saturated. In butter it is the result of bacterial action on unsaturated plant oils in the rumen of the cow. In food industry fats are the result of bubbling hydrogen through unsaturated vegetable and marine oils. The result is the same. All solid fats are better avoided as far as possible. Much better alternatives are available.

Use of Tropical Oils

The food industry uses saturated coconut, palm and palm kernel oils for many products, including cakes, pastries, biscuits, non-dairy creamers, confectionery and the like. Polyunsaturated oils and fats could be used instead.

CARBOHYDRATE

The first step is to reduce the amount of energy obtained from fat and increase that from carbohydrate, except for sugar, and especially from the nutritious starchy foods which include bread and other cereals, and potatoes.

The second step is to switch from white bread and other refined cereals to wholemeal bread and other *un*refined cereals, including the breakfast varieties.

Sugar has no nutritional value. It is best not to add sugar as a routine at table or in cooking, but to use it as an occasional spice when the flavour of food is definitely improved. Sugar makes a major contribution to obesity and dental decay. A 'sweet-tooth' is usually acquired early in life, and so sugar, like salt, is best not offered to infants and young children.

It is noteworthy that a high consumption of carbohydrate is associated with a low mortality from CHD, as seen in Japan and the Mediterranean countries.

Wholemeal Bread

Wholemeal bread is excellent nutritious food. The recommendation to eat 'five or six slices a day' is soundly based. If breakfast and a snack type lunch are included, it is easily done. By contrast, the bleached white variety of bread is, overall, an inferior substitute which has been deprived of bran, essential fatty acids and most of the minerals, vitamins and micronutrients.

There is still much to be learned about many nutrients, but there is no doubt that appreciable losses occur as more and more of the outer layers of the grain are removed in the milling process. A Medical Research Council Committee concluded that, 'the consumption of a 70% extraction (white) flour, even if it is partly fortified, would lead to a reduced intake of some nutrients. Although such a reduction would not necessarily lead to an increase in recognisable illness, it would, in the present state of knowledge, constitute a risk which can be avoided'. To this can now be added more about the value of cereal fibre.

Bread continues to be one of the world's important staple foods. The decline in consumption in affluent populations, which is encouraged by the poor quality of bread in the U.K., is to be deplored. There are sound reasons why children from an early age should be brought up on wholemeal bread rather than white. This should of course be cheaper because of the profit made by the industry in selling the germ and bran to fatten animals. This is one of many areas where the DHSS could exert some influence.

Dietary Fibre

Fibre is present in all unprocessed plant food, but there is none in food of animal origin. By absorbing water, fibre increases food bulk and helps to satisfy the appetite at low calorie cost and to maintain normal intestinal function. 'Swellability' has been graded and is greatest with bran, cauliflower, sprouts, apples and oranges. Western diets tend to be low in fibre because of the high consumption of refined carbohydrate and low intake of vegetables, cereals, fruit and nuts. The consequences include constipation, diverticular disease, spastic disorders of the colon, appendicitis, haemorrhoids, varicose veins and probably a contribution to cancer of the bowel.

Increasing Dietary Fibre: Oatmeal, pulses and apples have the advantage of reducing blood cholesterol concentrations. Carrots are also useful in supplying vitamin A. Green leafy vegetables also supply vitamin A and are an important source of the essential polyunsaturated fatty acids. Vitamin A is likely to have some protective effect against cancer.

CHILDREN

Developing tissues are the most susceptible to dietary injury and have the greatest requirements for nutrients. Atherosclerosis may be quite advanced in young adults and frequently starts in childhood. Pathological changes in the coronary arteries are by no means uncommon in children.[6,7] Pesonen in Helsinki has reported a large series with substantial (microscopical) changes even on the first day of life.[8] No matter what the cause, and there may be a number, it is to be expected that injury would normally be followed by repair, given a favourable nutritional environment. Under adverse circumstances, once the endothelial barrier is breached, the stage is set for atherosclerosis. It has been shown that hypercholesterolaemia itself may cause endothelial injury.

Correct maternal feeding during pregnancy as a preparation for breast feeding could be the first step in coronary prevention.

At present most children have a diet of similar composition to that of adults, which is to say it is potentially atherogenic, although there is likely to be varying individual susceptibility.

Food preferences and eating habits learned early are those most likely to be continued in later years. Children are much influenced by example and prevention is best regarded as a family affair.

In both the U.K. working party reports it was specifically stated that the dietary recommendations are relevant to children.

It follows that there is no nutritional sense in offering children butter or any other hydrogenated fat as a table spread, or to use anything other than polyunsaturated margarines and oils for cooking. If this were done in the home and was the usual practice in the school catering services, there need be no concern about 'eating out' because the overall contribution would be small. School meals are in urgent need of review.

Beyond reasonable doubt, the answer to the coronary problem starts in childhood with true primary prevention against atherosclerosis and the risk factors which lead to it.

WHOSE RESPONSIBILITY?

Present-day food policy is unrelated to nutrition. This is reflected in the

Government White Paper on Prevention and Health (1977)[9] in which it is stated that, 'The total pattern of demand for food representing the sum of individual choices freely made by members of the public should determine food policy'. Several points should be noted.

First, freedom of choice is largely a myth. This is partly due to government action, or inaction, usually for political reasons or in deference to powerful vested interests which, on their own admission, have little or no interest in health except insofar as food should be safe in the conventional sense. Examples of interference are subsidies and taxes on foods, or support systems affecting producer price and favouring, for example, fat carcases, full-fat milk and butter. Although the DHSS have advised a reduction in the consumption of saturated fat, to which dairy fat makes by far the largest single contribution, MAFF has subsidised butter with a view to increasing consumption on account of the European 'mountain'. This is paradoxical to say the least.

Absence of informative labelling or the presence of labelling which is misleading also restricts free choice. It is not possible to know the fat content of cheese, sausages and numerous other products, or the fatty acid composition of margarine. Price is an important consideration for many, and yet it is often manipulated primarily to benefit the producer.

Unfettered advertising of foods influences consumption in directions against the recommendations of doctors, nutritionists and the DHSS.

The dairy industry is permitted to spend £12 million in a single year promoting full-fat dairy produce, specifically aimed at the young. By contrast, nutritional education to counter the efforts of the food industry is inadequate. A relative pittance is given to the Health Education Council.

The government says, 'its responsibilities should be directed primarily to assembling, assessing and disseminating information based on scientific evidence in the light of which individuals can form their own views and take their own decisions'. There are fundamental misconceptions here. Reference has already been made to the myth of freedom of choice. Next it must be emphasised that the public has *not* been well informed by the DHSS or anyone else. Despite claims made, none of the official booklets, even the latest *Eating for Health*, is up to date or in any sense a discussion document. In this area the DHSS lacks authority. They have not obviously influenced MAFF or the government in formulating a food policy linked to health. The necessary structure for implementing the recommendations for a more prudent diet or of co-ordinating the many activities related to a nutritional policy does not exist in the U.K. Six years after publication in 1974 of a report by the DHSS Committee on Medical Aspects of Food (COMA) on Diet and Coronary Heart Disease,[10] no change has resulted. They take the view that prevention is 'Everbody's Business', but few are sufficiently well informed, freedom of choice is largely a myth and prices are manipulated to suit the producer. The COMA report was not sent to doctors nor were circulars sent to Area Health Authorities as would have been expected. Likewise, the report was not sent to food producers, manufacturers or to caterers. School meals, hospital meals and institutional meals are unchanged.

There is clearly need for a Central Authority at Ministerial level to co-ordinate government departments. There could be a Minister of Food in overall charge of a committee with Ministers of Agriculture and of Food Manufacturer, of Nutrition, of Education and Ministers or representatives concerned with the problems of the EEC, of imports, prices, advertising, labelling and so on.

It is time for a change. The responsibility for preventive medicine lies primarily with the government. In a recent address to a Conference on Smoking and Health, a Junior Minister in the DHSS said that, 'The solution to many of today's medical problems will not be found in research laboratories, but in our Parliaments. For the prospective patient the answer may not be cured by incision at the operating table, but prevention by decision at the Cabinet table. If you look at most of the big killer diseases of today, they are not caused by nature, but by our way of life. They include heart attacks, strokes, cancer and road accidents. The answer to these illnesses is not cure, but prevention, and does not raise medical issues, but political ones, since it predisposes the adjustment of a nation's lifestyle to improve itself. Historically a nation would look to its doctors for better health. Now they should look to their Members of Parliament. There is growing evidence of the willingness of Parliaments throughout the world to legislate to protect an individual from damaging his own health. The cost of illness may not be borne by the individual, but through our NHS by tax payers as a whole'.

CONCLUSION

It is becoming widely agreed that what is required is commitment by governments to preventive medicine. It is clear that in the long run there will in effect have to be new agricultural and food industrial revolutions, but changes are bound to be gradual and this will allow for adaptation.

Continuing inaction amounts to condoning a man-made epidemic, the answer to which lies in man's hands. The risks of CHD are known and large, but those of the proposed action are little or hypothetical.

Scotland now shares with Finland the highest mortality from CHD in the world, and England and Wales are not far behind. The reasons are not far to seek. There will be no spontaneous improvement in this serious situation and action is demanded. Is further evidence required before action?

There can be no 'proof' of any dietary theory by dietary trials owing to the long incubation period of the underlying arterial disease before symptoms develop. Significantly stronger evidence could not possibly be established in the foreseeable future, nor is it considered necessary. For the same reason significantly better prediction of those at high risk who alone need be given preventive advice could not be established by further research.

For practical purposes in the U.K., the whole population must be considered at risk since most have atherosclerosis. At present there is no non-invasive technique for monitoring its development and progression. It is known to be widespread and is often severe in the apparently healthy, and so prevention must be directed at the population as a whole.

What matters is not greater certainty, but a decision on acceptable levels of risk, and this is a socio-political matter. Since literal proof is unobtainable, 'proof' for practical purposes amounts to probability.

REFERENCES

(1) U.S. Nat. Inst. Hlth., 'Arteriosclerosis, a report by the National Heart & Lung Institute Task Force on Arteriosclerosis' 1, *DHEW Pub. No.* (NH) 72 (1971).

(2) H. Blackburn, B. Lewis, R.W. Wissler *et al.,* "Conference on the health effects of blood lipids: optimal distributions for populations" *Prev. Med.* 8, 612 (1979).

(3) R.W. Wissler, D. Vesselinovitch, R. Hughes *et al,* "Atherosclerosis and blood lipids in rhesus monkeys fed human table-prepared diets" *Circ.* 44, suppl. 2, 57 (1971).

(4) R.W. Wissler and D. Vesselinovitch, "Comparative pathogenetic patterns in atherosclerosis" *Adv. Lipid Res.* 6, 181 (1968).

(5) R.W. Wissler and D. Vesselinovitch, "Atherosclerosis in non-human primates" *Adv. Vet. Sci. Comp. Med.* 21, 351 (1977).

(6) G.R. Osborn, *Incubation Period of Coronary Thrombosis* 1963 (Butterworths, London, 1973) p. 177.

(7) G.R. Osborn, "Stages in development of coronary heart disease observed from 1,500 young subjects" (Editions du centre national de la recherche scientifique, Paris, 1968) No. 169.

(8) E. Pesonen, "Coronary wall thickening in children" *Atherosclerosis* 20, 173 (1974).

(9) *Prevention and Health,* Govt. White Paper (HMSO, London, 1977).

(10) Department of Health & Social Security (COMA), *Diet and Coronary Heart Disease* (HMSO, London, 1974).

-5-

Essential
Trace Mineral Deficiencies
and Cardiovascular Disease

Dennis Shapcott

SUMMARY

At least 6 elements present in trace amounts in body tissue and in food have been shown to be essential for normal health in humans. Although there is no evidence to support the hypothesis that trace element deficiency of itself is the etiologic factor in the development of atherosclerotic cardiac disease, experimental studies on animals and epidemiologic and clinical studies on humans indicate that chromium deficiency is probably and copper deficiency possibly associated with worsening of the risk factors for ACD.

For many years the existence of major differences between different countries in the morbidity of atherosclerotic cardiovascular disease (ACD) has been beyond dispute. The fact that people migrating from a low incidence country to a high incidence country tend to develop ACD in the same manner as their new fellow countrymen eliminates an explanation of the greater morbidity on purely genetic grounds. Much research has been devoted, therefore, in an effort to identify metabolic factors which could be implicated in ACD. From this research, several "risk factors" have been defined, originally because of their higher incidence in ACD, and subsequently to explain the formation of the atherosclerotic plaques believed to be the initiating factor in ACD. Among these metabolic risk factors which appear to have stood the test of time are hypercholesterolemia, decrease in high density lipoprotein, reduced glucose tolerance and, more recently hyperinsulinemia. It would not be appropriate at this time to evaluate the significance of these risk factors in relation to ACD, but instead to consider how trace mineral deficiency could result in their production.

DIET AND ACD

One outstanding difference between low and high ACD incidence countries lies in their dietary practices. High incidence subjects eat diets relatively rich in animal protein with the bulk of their calories from fat (mostly animal fat) and refined carbohydrate including simple sugars. Contrariwise, low incidence subjects eat mostly unrefined vegetable products with little animal fat or protein. As a result, much effort has been spent in demonstrating that an *excess* of sucrose, cholesterol, animal fat or animal protein provokes atherosclerosis but apart from the possibility that our diet lacks essential polyunsaturated fatty acids, little attempt has been made to identify nutritional *deficiencies* in the development of ACD. This is even more so in the case of the minor nutritional components with the possible exception of vitamin E. However, in recent years the attempts to define the metabolic roles of the essential trace elements have shown that differences exist in the minor dietary components between low and high ACD incidence countries which are as significant as those occurring between the fats, proteins and carbohydrates.

In a review in 1978, Klevay[1] listed 29 elements which had been associated either with ACD or with derangements in lipid metabolism (Table I). This list included the macroelements such as sodium and potassium, certain microelements normally considered to be toxic and also those known to be essential for normal health. Since changes in sodium and potassium metabolism represent alterations in their homeostatic regulation rather than dietary deficiencies, and since sulphur as the element plays no role in human metabolism our attention must be directed towards the minor dietary constituents, the trace elements. Of the 24 elements in Klevay's list that are present in trace quantities in human tissues and in the dietary intake, 11 are considered to be toxic and metabolic functions for them have not yet been defined.[2]

Table I: Elements Associated with Ischemic Heart Disease

Macroelements	Toxic Trace Elements	Essential Trace Elements
Calcium	Antimony	Arsenic
Magnesium	Cadmium	Chromium
Potassium	Cerium	Cobalt
Sodium	Germanium	Copper
Sulphur	Indium	Fluorine
	Lead	Iodine
	Lithium	Iron
	Mercury	Manganese
	Niobium	Molybdenum
	Tellurium	Nickel
	Zirconium	Selenium
		Tin
		Zinc

THE ESSENTIAL TRACE ELEMENTS

In the absence of an entirely satisfactory definition, essential trace elements may be defined for our purpose as those elements essential for health whose circulating levels are in the nanomolar to micromolar range.

Trace element research historically was directed toward animal husbandry in order to alleviate certain metabolic defects arising from the consumption of plants grown on mineral-deficient or mineral-rich soil. Our knowledge of the metabolic effects of trace elements is thus far greater for animals than for man, and it is only in very recent years that this knowledge has been applied to human health.

Trace element essentially may be defined at three levels of confidence.

(1) A defined pathology occurring in humans which is prevented by supplementation with the trace element.

(2) The development of a pathological condition in animals fed a diet deficient in a specific trace element which condition is ameliorated by supplementation with the trace element.

(3) Demonstration that a trace element is a cofactor for an enzyme essential in human metabolism.

Obviously, the first definition is the most satisfactory but most of our knowledge has been obtained using the technique of the second definition. This has produced much confusion, since the effects of trace element deficiencies, like those of vitamin deficiencies, vary greatly between different genera and in many cases, such as vitamin E deficiency in rats and rabbits, do not resemble any pathological condition described in man.

A further point of confusion is that many of the effects ascribed to trace element have been produced by inducing a deficiency in the growing animal and so little is known of the effects of deficiency developing in the adult.[3]

It must be remembered, however, that although ACD manifests itself in later life, the plaques believed to be the precursors of the atherosclerotic process are present in young adults and even infants and so the precipitating factors for ACD are present during childhood; thus trace element deficiency in early life may predispose to the subsequent development of ACD.

From Table I it can be seen that 13 trace elements are essential to mammals; of these 6 fulfil the criterion of the first definition above with a definite pathology associated with deficiency (Table II).

Table II: Trace Elements Where Deficiency Is Associated with Definite Pathology in Man*

Element	Deficiency State
Chromium	Diabetes mellitus
Copper	Anemia
Fluorine	Dental caries
Iodine	Goitre
Iron	Anemia
Zinc	Dermatoses, dwarfism

*Cobalt has not been included since there is no evidence that the metal itself plays any role in human metabolism.

In this paper I shall review the epidemiological, experimental and clinical evidence that indicates a role for trace element deficiencies as risk factors in the development of ACD.

EPIDEMIOLOGICAL EVIDENCE

Hard Versus Soft Water

An inverse relationship between ACD and the hardness of drinking water has been noted by investigators in several countries.

In the U.S., Canada, Britain, Sweden and the Netherlands investigators have reported an inverse correlation between ACD morbidity and mortality, and water hardness.[4-8] This, of itself, leads to two opposing conclusions, namely that the hard water contains substances missing from the soft water which are necessary for normal health, or alternatively, that soft water, being a much better solvent could contain toxic substances (e.g., cadmium) which have been dissolved from pipes or metal fittings. Only the first possibility will be discussed here.

Hard water contains anions, phosphate and silicate, often chloride and as major cations calcium and magnesium with varying amounts of sodium and potassium and trace metals both essential and toxic at very low concentration (Table III).

Table III: Essential Mineral Content of Potable Water from the Largest Cities of the U.S.

Macroelements	Range, mg/ℓ	Microelements	Range, μg/ℓ
Calcium	0.3-92	Chromium	0-35
Fluorine	0-2.5	Copper	0.61-237
Magnesium	0.02-35	Iron	4.8-1,000
Potassium	0-9.2	Manganese	0-154
Sodium	1.1-119	Molybdenum	0-16
		Nickel	0-34
		Vanadium	0-28

Source: Schroeder, Reference 4

From this table it is evident that even for those waters with the greatest mineral content, one litre of water would supply only a small fraction of the daily requirements (excepting possibly chromium and manganese).

It is apparent that the wide range of concentration makes it most difficult to assess the possibility of an effect due to any one of the constituents from this evidence alone. In view of the central roles of calcium and magnesium in muscle metabolism, these two metals have been most frequently implicated, and most authors have postulated magnesium as the target factor since calcium is present in far greater amounts in foodstuffs; also, the absorption of calcium being regulated by hormonal factors, it is unlikely that a deficiency could arise in soft water subjects on the sole grounds of somewhat reduced intake.

Anderson has shown decreased levels of magnesium (but not other metals) in the myocardium from soft water subjects as compared with hard water;[9] lower calcium and magnesium levels in the arteries were found in subjects from soft water areas in the U.K.[10]

The conclusion that magnesium deficiency can arise from drinking soft water is open to criticism on the grounds that for the hardest water in Schroeder's study, one litre would contribute only 15% of the daily requirement, probably much of this water would be taken as hot beverages when the magnesium is precipitated as scale by heating, similarly water used for the manufacture of beverages is usually demineralised. It seems unlikely that the absence of a source for a few percent of the daily intake would result in deficiency, above all since absorption of magnesium (like some other metals) becomes more effective with lower intake. A more likely possibility is that the relative deficiency in myocardial magnesium is secondary to other metabolic factors. In this regard, Stitt reported elevated blood pressure and serum cholesterol in a soft water area, but there is no evidence that magnesium was implicated.[11]

A recent study in Finland has shown low serum zinc levels (but normal serum copper levels) in subjects living in areas of old rock with low mineral content of surface water.[12] Although zinc deficiency has not been implicated as a causal factor in ACD, nevertheless this study shows that trace metal deficiency can occur due to low levels in potable water.

In another study reported from Finland, the rate of ACD morbidity was shown to be inversely related to the chromium content of drinking water.[13]

It is conceptually difficult to associate ACD with low levels of minerals in drinking water since normally these do not comprise a significant part of the daily intake (Table III). However it may be possible that with deficient intake from other sources, then drinking water could become the limiting factor.

Trace Element Deficiency

There has been great interest in ACD in Finland both since that country has the highest morbidity and mortality and also since the distribution of ACD varies greatly within the country. In the search for a metabolic factor to account for this situation it has been shown that the circulating levels of selenium are considerably lower in that country than in other Western countries.[14] So far it has not proven possible to associate this directly with ACD, although as will be mentioned, selenium deficiency could be a precipitating factor. It has also recently been shown that the circulating selenium level in a representative population in New Zealand was also much lower than elsewhere.[15] The incidence of CHD is no greater there than in other Western countries, however.

Tissue levels of chromium have been shown to be lower in autopsy material from the U.S. than in other countries, particularly the lesser developed countries.[16] Furthermore, the tissue levels in humans were lower than those found in domestic or wild animals giving further proof that the subjects were in fact, deficient in chromium. These findings are in agreement with fact that the chromium content of foodstuffs is lower in the more highly refined ingredients used in Western countries, for example, the use of refined sugar instead of the complex carbohydrate consumed by most of the world's population.[17] The chromium content of different nutritionally adequate diets may vary from 5 to 115 μg/day, so that very low intakes of the metal are possible.[18] The total chromium content of representative diets has varied from 130-280 μg/day in Canada[19-20], 455-887 μg/day in hospital menus in the U.S.[21], 60 μg/day in the U.S. and lower values in New Zealand.[22] As always, the reliability of measurement of chromium at these levels was probably marginal and these values are almost certainly much too high. However, a caveat must be entered to the effect that the intestinal absorption of chromium (as with other trace minerals) is greatly influenced by its chemical form and therefore measure of total chromium intake can only give the maximum possible absorption.[23] It is also unclear if, as is the case with iron, there is a regulatory mechanism at the level of the enterocyte, which controls absorption. Chromium is unique among the essential trace metals in that it is excreted mostly by the kidney. Recent reports indicate a loss of about 10-20 μg/day in normal subjects; this presumably represents the actual absorption of the metal.[24]

It has also been proposed by Klevay, that the daily copper intake in North America is marginal at best and that borderline and low level deficiency is prevalent among the apparently healthy population.[25] This is difficult to confirm, particularly in the light of the ubiquity of this element and the high possibility of intake other than the actual ingredients of food (use of copper utensils, copper piping etc. . .). A low intake of copper has also been suggested by others[26-27] although in a balance study carried out on normal subjects taking representative diets there was a slight positive retention of the metal.[28] An intake of 2 mg/day is considered necessary as the recommended daily allowance in the U.S., and it appears that most people do not obtain this amount from food.

In summary although the difference in ACD mortality between subjects living in hard water and soft water areas may be attributed to minerals in the water it is far from clear which minerals could be involved. Foodstuffs from high ACD areas have lower content of certain trace minerals, particularly chromium, copper, and selenium but whether this means that the population of high ACD countries must be deficient in these elements remains a moot point.

EVIDENCE FROM EXPERIMENTAL STUDIES

Although ACD does not occur naturally in those animals from whom our knowledge of the metabolic activities of the trace elements has been obtained, nevertheless, by dietary manipulations syndromes resembling ACD may be produced or risk aggravated (Table IV).

Cobalt–The only known metabolic function of cobalt is as vitamin B_{12} in two reactions–the isomerisation of methylmalonic acid (MMA) and reformation of methionine from cysteine. Cobalt deficiency is a lethal condition in ruminants resulting in the production of large quantities of propionic acid–the precursor of MMA. It is not known if animals, ruminants excepted, have a specific need for cobalt other than as vitamin B_{12}.

Copper–This element participates in several reactions as a cofactor for oxidases and two of these in particular, cytochrome oxidase and lysyl oxidase could be implicated in ACD, the former enzyme by virtue of its central role in the production of energy within the cell. Lysyl oxidase functions in the production of crosslinks in collagen which serve to stabilise this protein, and copper deficiency in growing animals results in defective collagen formation in the aorta with obvious physical defects in the vessel.[29] Desaturation of fatty acids by microsomal oxidase was reduced in copper-deficient rats. This could have implications for phospholipid metabolism and membrane structure, both of which play a part in the atherosclerotic process.

Table IV: The Biological Activity of Elements Necessary for Normal Health*

Element	Biological Activity
Chromium	Glucose metabolism, insulin activity
Cobalt	Only as vitamin B_{12}
Copper	Component of oxidase enzymes, biosynthesis of haem, collagen biosynthesis
Fluorine	Increases physical resistance of dentine and bone
Iodine	Thyroid hormones
Iron	Haem proteins, iron-sulphur proteins
Manganese	Glucose metabolism
Molybdenum	Xanthine oxidase, interacts with copper and sulphate
Nickel	Growth-specific activity not known
Selenium	Glutathione peroxidase
Silicon	Collagen biosynthesis
Tin	Necessary for normal growth
Vanadium	Glucose metabolism
Zinc	Connective tissue integrity, immune response, many others

*For most elements, the function at the molecular level is not yet defined; in many cases, e.g., tin, nickel, the metabolic pathways involved are as yet unknown.

Of considerable interest is the report from Klevay that dietary supplementation with zinc in animals results in decreased serum copper levels and increased serum cholesterol.[30] However, at least two other reports have appeared since showing no effect on the serum cholesterol level even with 30-fold increase in the Zn/Cu ratio.[31,32] The reasons for the discrepancy between these reports are not evident and the significance of the original findings must remain in doubt.

Copper has not been shown to be a cofactor in the biosynthesis of cholesterol, and so presumably any effect on plasma cholesterol level is due to alteration in cholesterol homeostasis, such as decreased bile salt synthesis or decreased biliary excretion.

Manganese is intimately involved in glucose tolerance and deficiency in experimental animals results in impaired glucose tolerance and intracellular fat deposition.[33] The molecular mechanisms responsible have not yet been elucidated but impaired energy metabolism and abnormal lipid metabolism evidently can be implicated as factors in the atherosclerotic process. Manganese also participates in the glucosyl transferase reactions involved in the biosynthesis of connective tissue.[34]

Chromium was shown by Schwartz and Mertz to be a component of a substance present in brewers' yeast which is essential for normal glucose tolerance (the glucose tolerance factor, GTF).[35] Studies on chromium may be classified either as whole animal studies or those carried out on isolated tissues. In the whole animal studies, chromium deficiency induced by dietary deficiency has resulted in decreased glucose tolerance in several species of animals.[36,37] Given a severe chronic deficiency the animals may develop a frankly diabetic state.[38] Old breeder rats put on a chromium-deficient diet rapidly develop an almost complete resistance to exogenous insulin.[39]

Animals which had received supplemental chromium showed increased longevity, lower serum cholesterol levels and fewer aortic plaques than control animals.[40,41] It is of considerable interest that, in general, male animals appeared to be more sensitive to the effects of chromium deficiency and supplementation than did female animals. There is a certain species difference also in the effects of chromium deficiency since squirrel monkeys develop cataracts while rats and rabbits do not.

A factor of great importance in considering the biological activity of this metal is its chemical state. Inorganic chromium salts are poorly absorbed and also appear to have little effect upon isolated tissue cells in vitro.[42,43] It appears that the chromium must be in the form of a GTF or chemically similar complex both for absorption and for biological activity in tissue.[44]

Vanadium can be considered to play a role in the regulation of glucose metabolism since vanadates act synergistically with insulin in increasing glucose transport and oxidation in isolated cells.[45] Little is known, however, of its function in vivo.

Selenium, originally considered to be a toxic element, is now known to be essential for health in mammals. This element is remarkable for the narrow range from lethal deficiency to toxic excess.[2] So far its only metabolic function is as part of the enzyme glutathione peroxidase, which plays a key role in the detoxification of the free radicles and peroxides formed within the cell during normal metabolism.[46] Evidently, decreased activity of this enzyme could result in cellular degeneration; in fact selenium deficiency causes a fatal liver necrosis in rats, but induced deficiencies in animals are not specifically associated with the changes in blood vessels found in ACD.[47]

Molybdenum evidences no correlation with ACD in experimental animals and the sole function ascribed to the metal at the molecular level is as cofactor for the enzymes xanthine oxidase, aldehyde oxidase and sulfite oxidase.[48] However, as discussed below, Mo may participate in an indirect manner in cholesterol metabolism.

Of the more recently described essential trace minerals, *silicon* has been implicated in collagen metabolism,[49] but as with *nickel* and *tin* so little is known about their physiological and molecular functions that there is insufficient data base to form any hypothesis.

Trace Mineral Interactions

Much interest is developing in the effect of the interaction between the trace minerals upon their metabolic activities. Since the chemical activity of an atom is due to its electronic structure, and since there are numerous examples –particularly among the transition elements–of elements which are isoelectronic for the electrons in their outer shells, then one can postulate certain specific interactions.

Furthermore, interactions involving more than two elements are known to occur, such as the copper-molybdenum-sulphate, this particular interaction being of practical importance in ruminant health.[50]

In animal experiments several elements have been shown to interact antagonistically, including manganese-iron, zinc-copper and vanadium-chromium. These latter two pairs are germane to our theme, and demonstrate that the consideration of single elements in isolation is too simplistic an approach and, particularly in epidemiological studies of trace mineral metabolism a multifactorial approach should be adopted.[51]

In summary, evidence from experimental studies indicates a strong possibility that deficiency of chromium is associated with worsening of risk factors and thus with development of ACD; the evidence that copper is thus associated remains equivocal.

CLINICAL STUDIES IN HUMANS

While much information has been obtained from studies where the dietary intake has been modified for macronutients such as fatty acids, sugars and starches and proteins, there is little information concerning the effect of supplementation with trace minerals.

It is obvious that the type of experiment which has furnished our knowledge thus far–the induction of deficiency in animals by the use of artificial diets with observation of the development of pathological symptoms–cannot be carried out in humans. Instead, recourse is made to retrospective studies to determine the probability of deficiency in certain pathological conditions and the amelioration resulting from trace mineral supplementation. This latter may be difficult to assess since ethical considerations must preclude the withholding of other therapies so that synergistic or antagonistic effects due to drugs will occur.

Measurement of Trace Element Levels

It is only within the past few years that methods with sensitivity and precision adequate for the measurement of micronutrients in foods, body tissues and body fluids have become available. It is obvious from the case of chromium that little credence can be placed on the results from studies carried out before this decade.

In a recent comprehensive review, Versieck shows that even among experienced analysts using identical techniques there is little agreement on what constitutes normal values for trace elements in plasma in healthy subjects.[52] Because of this there is little point in comparing values between different laboratories and so most investigators prefer to compare changes in trace element levels as result of induced metabolic variation, or to compare an index population with a healthy control population.

It appears most logical to consider trace element levels in terms of "concentration windows".[2] Dietary intakes below a certain level result in disease from deficiency while values above a different level are associated with disease from excess. The range between (the concentration window) is thus associated with health; this range for selenium in the rat is very narrow, but is considerably wider for iron, and iron is thus considered to be less toxic.

In general, the major difference between "essential" and "toxic" trace minerals is that the concentration window is wider for the former because of the higher levels necessary for toxic effects. It is difficult to induce toxic tissue levels of essential trace minerals by dietary manipulations although the difference between essentiality and toxicity is decreasing, as witness the recent definition of arsenic as trace mineral.[53]

This same logic can be applied to levels in blood and tissue. Hence, it is more appropriate to obviate the use of means and standard deviations and to consider as abnormal those values which fall below the lowest values found in healthy subjects, or perhaps, more realistically, those values below or in the same range as the lowest 10th percentile of a healthy population. There is now enough data available to state unequivocally that trace element levels vary with age and sometimes with sex, which is obviously an important factor in considering a possible association with ACD.

Tissue and Body Fluids: Even given satisfactory analytical techniques the definition of trace mineral deficiency poses many problems. The overriding problem of sample contamination necessitates such extreme measures as the collection of blood via a plastic catheter into a specially acid washed container since the containers used normally for this purpose are hopelessly contaminated. Collection of urine, food and tissue samples, while less difficult than blood samples still requires far greater precaution against contamination than for more conventional analyses.[54] Indeed, it is probable that the differing values which are currently reported from different laboratories are due to sample contamination rather than differences in analytical precision.

The actual demonstration of trace element deficiency is far from satisfactory for the elements under discussion here. Perhaps the most widely studied of these is zinc, and the methods utilised can serve as an illustration. Zinc is present in tissues and body fluids at comparatively high levels (in parts per million) so that analysis is straightforward and there is general agreement as to the plasma zinc levels (collected under standard conditions) from healthy subjects. However, there is a diurnal variation in plasma zinc levels,[55] and the value varies greatly following a meal; the normal range is wide. In some subjects with symptoms attributable to zinc deficiency and who responded to zinc supplementation the plasma levels were not significantly below normal levels[56] and at present it seems that while acute severe deficiency results in definitely abnormal plasma levels this is not necessarily so with chronic mild deficiency. Zinc deficiency may be due to increased urinary loss of the metal and thus a considerable increase in urine zinc level would be presumptive evidence of a deficient state.[57]

Most of the trace metals are actively secreted into the growing hair and remain fixed there; in most cases the hair level is much greater than the plasma level. Hair zinc has been used as an index of deficiency, and in at least one study correlated well with the clinical condition.[58] An objection to hair analysis is that it must be purely retrospective, and so the slow growth of hair makes it unsatisfactory as an immediate measure of acute deficiency.

Saliva has been suggested as an analytical medium for trace mineral determination both on the grounds that collection is simple and the level of the particular element may represent a "free" (non-protein-bound) biologically active form.[59] However, at present little is known concerning the relationship between tissue levels and saliva levels.

The most satisfactory means of evaluation is a metabolic balance whereby intake and output can be measured and thus the body uptake can be calculated, although this obviously requires that the test subject be studied in a metabolic unit, which limits its availability. As a modification of this technique the uptake of radioactive zinc by erythrocytes *in vitro* has been proposed on the grounds that deficient subjects will have lower erythrocyte levels, and will thus take up more of the labelled zinc.[60] This approach may be justified for zinc which has a well-defined role in the erythrocyte (and high levels also) but for the other metals such a role has not been demonstrated.

Trace Element Levels in Food: Nutritional deficiencies have been defined as intake less than the Recommended Daily Allowance (RDA), this being the amount necessary for the maintenance of health. This approach forms the basis for the "dietary goals for the United States" which has been criticised by Harper[61] on the grounds that the following assumptions: "(1) that the United States is suffering from an epidemic of chronic degenerative diseases; (2) that alterations in the composition of the food supply during the 20th century are in some way responsible for the high incidence of chronic degenerative diseases; and (3) that modification of the food supply and of the American diet generally is an appropriate and effective measure for reducing the incidence of, and death rates from, these diseases"—may be invalid. Furthermore, the rationale for dietary intervention will vary according to the objective i.e., to maintain good health or to reduce the incidence of certain degenerative diseases. In the first case the daily intake of an element by the general population is evidently adequate; for the second objective the intake may have to be increased.

The absorption of a mineral varies greatly according to its chemical form—for example the absorption of Cr as the oxalate is an order of magnitude greater than that of the chloride.[62] A further factor is the presence of phytate, nonabsorbable fibre and excess phsophate which tend to decrease absorption by the formation of insoluble complexes, while the presence of other trace minerals can change the absorption of a specific element in a positive or negative manner.

Although six years have passed since the above criteria were proposed the situation has not changed markedly and much more data is needed before

RDA's can confidently be ascribed to the trace minerals. In general it would appear that the dietary intake in the U.S. and Canada (and probably in most Western countries) is marginally adequate at best for chromium; and for the other essential microelements the daily requirements are not yet established. It does not appear, however, that there is a great risk of developing deficiencies in the minor trace elements such as vanadium, molybdenum, etc. . .

Trace Element Levels in Blood and Tissue: A number of reports have appeared describing changes in trace element levels in blood and tissue in ACD and in diabetes. In some of these, e.g., the finding by Sunderman of an acute increase in the serum nickel following myocardial infarct, there is no obvious association with the development of ACD.[63] This is also true of the studies by Nazdryukhina who reported differences in a number of trace elements in subjects with ACD.[64]

The general weakness of such studies is that unless some correlation is made with an appropriate physiological parameter–such as glucose tolerance or serum cholesterol–then the significance of deviations in trace element levels must remain speculative.

From the reasons cited above, it appears that chromium, and to a lesser extent copper may be implicated in ACD so only these will be considered here.

Copper–Klevay's reports of a negative correlation between serum copper and serum cholesterol in rats have sparked interest in the possibility that hypercholesterolemia in humans may be associated with copper deficiency. There have been contradictory reports on the effect of zinc supplementation on serum copper levels; in two studies on healthy elderly subjects there was no relationship between zinc intake and copper levels.[65,66]

Three more recent studies on long-term supplementation with zinc in Down's syndrome and sickle cell disease have shown a decrease in serum copper,[67,68] and also in normal subjects.[69] It would appear thus that with massive zinc supplementation (10 times the normal daily intake) copper deficiency may be induced but this is not likely to occur simply by changes in the dietary intake. It is unfortunate that the serum cholesterol was not measured in these studies to determine how great a change in copper levels is necessary to produce hypercholesterolemia. This is obviously a subject of considerable practical importance in view of the ever-increasing use of zinc supplementation for specific medical problems, also its use with vitamins as a dietary supplement in healthy subjects.

Insofar as copper levels in ACD is concerned both low and high values have been reported, while increased levels in serum and urine were found in diabetes mellitus.

Chromium–The literature is replete with contradictory findings regarding tissue and blood chromium levels in different disorders.

Schroeder and Tipton reported lower chromium levels in aortas from Americans as compared with subjects from the Third World countries and lower levels in Americans dying from ACD than in those dying from accidents.[70] Morgan reported lower liver chromium levels in diabetics but this was not confirmed by Eatough in his study on Pima Indians.[71]

In considering blood and urine chromium levels, the older studies must be suspect because of the very high levels found. If we consider those studies within the past 10 years, there has been almost continuous decline in reported values and there is still no general agreement as to what constitutes normal values even amongst workers using the same analytical techniques. To illustrate this problem, there is a greater than 50-fold variation in the reported values for serum chromium levels as measured by atomic absorption spectroscopy. For this reason, most workers have preferred to measure the increment or decrement in serum chromium following a glucose challenge. One recent report, however, showed no difference in serum chromium between normal subjects and those with a history of myocardial infarct,[72] while another showed significantly lower serum chromium in subjects with ACD.[73] Insofar as changes in plasma chromium are concerned, most investigators agree that there is an increase in plasma chromium level in response to a glucose challenge.[74,75] This increase may be identical for diabetics and non-diabetics, or more usually shows a reciprocal relationship with blood glucose levels.

Urinary chromium levels also appear to be negatively related to serum glucose levels and thus the increase is greater in non-diabetic subjects.[76]

Hair has also been used as an analytical medium for chromium and offers the advantage that the hair chromium level is at least 3 orders of magnitude greater than serum or urine levels. Because of this, the problem of contamination during collection and sample processing is much less acute and there is far closer agreement among the individual investigators as to the reference values in healthy population (Table V).

Table V: Hair Chromium Levels
(ng Cr/g hair)

Normal Adults
   (a)[1] Range of means: 241-750 (females).
        Range of means: 240-1,030 (males).

   (b) Mean values: 175,[2] 240, 770[3] (males).
        Mean values: 221, 250[2] (females).

Normal Children
   (a)[4] Mean 1,039 at 12 months, 660 at 3 years.
   (b)[1] At birth 125, children 190-408.

Pregnancy
   (a)[5] 200 pregnant; 750 non-pregnant.
   (b)[6] 284 pregnant; 567 two years after delivery.
   (c)[1] 251 at delivery; 249 two months later.

Diabetes
   (a)[7] Children: 560 (control 850).
   (b)[3] Adult males: not different from control (770).
   (c)[2] Adult males: 240 (control 175).
   (d)[2] Adult females: 140 (control 250).

Malnourished Elderly Women
   (a)[8] 257 (controls 499).

(continued)

Footnotes to Table V

[1]From Saner, op.cit. (76), p. 60
[2]Reference 80
[3]Reference 81
[4]Reference 82
[5]Reference 83
[6]Reference 84
[7]Reference 85
[8]Reference 86

Note: The values from footnote 1 were obtained
from subjects in various countries; those
in footnote 2, from the U.K.; the rest, from
the U.S. and Canada.

The lower values have been found in diabetics and in pregnant women and it appears also that the values are greatest in early infancy, although it is not clear if there is a continuous decline during adult life. Lower levels are found in diabetics, and in one case only in female diabetics. In a group of males with ACD, although the mean hair chromium level was not significantly lower than in a control group, more of the ACD subjects had hair chromium levels in the lower percentile.[77]

The key regulatory enzyme for hepatic cholesterol synthesis, hydroxymethyl-glutaryl CoA is activated by insulin, and so from the data presented here on chromium in mammalian metabolism one can postulate a role for chromium deficiency in the pathogenesis of ACD (Table VI).

**Table VI: Postulated Role of Chromium Deficiency
in Pathogenesis of ACD**

Dietary Chromium Deficiency
↓
Hyperglycemia (Decreased Insulin Activity)
↓
Hyperinsulinemia
↓
Hypercholesterolemia

As chromium is necessary for insulin-mediated utilisation of glucose, then Cr deficiency will lead to intolerance to glucose with concomitant hypersecretion of insulin, resulting in hypercholesterolemia. Thus worsening of 3 risk factors for ACD can be due to chromium deficiency.

SUPPLEMENTATION WITH CHROMIUM

Following the discovery of the glucose tolerance factor there was considerable interest in the possibility that chromium supplementation could improve glucose tolerance. The results for earlier trials can be summarised as follows—when a relatively high dose (1 mg) was given daily for 3 months to adult diabetics about a half showed improved glucose tolerance.[78] In the case of malnourished infants with impaired glucose tolerance this could be normalised following a single oral dose of chromic chloride.[79] The reasons for this difference in response between adult and infant is not clear—perhaps the adults have chronic deficiency which requires long-term supplementation or alternatively the infant may have a greater capacity to absorb the metal.

The low absorbability of inorganic chromium salts has provoked the use of preparations of brewers' yeast rich in glucose tolerance factor. Several studies have shown an improvement in glucose tolerance in diabetics and in older subjects following yeast supplementation, accompanied by a significant decline in serum insulin levels and in serum cholesterol. A most interesting finding was a decrease in serum cholesterol and insulin response to glucose following yeast in young subjects with normal glucose tolerance.[78]

A recent study of the effects of yeast supplementation on cholesterol and LDL and HDL cholesterol in a group of middle-aged men showed improvement by a decrease in LDL and concomitant increase in HDL after six weeks.[80]

While these results are most encouraging, yeast is a complex mixture of substances and so there is no definite proof that this effect was due only to GTF. While no one has yet succeeded in isolating the pure substance from yeast, there has been a recent report that chromium trisacetylacetonate is more readily absorbed than inorganic chromium salts and has high biological activity so this substance may provide an acceptable substitute for GTF.[87]

In Summary—From the available evidence[81-86] it appears that dietary chromium deficiency could play a role in the development of the atherosclerotic lesion both by derangement of energy metabolism and excessive cholesterogenesis. Copper deficiency may also be implicated on the grounds that this could result in hypercholesterolemia but the evidence for this occurring as a result of dietary modifications is not particularly strong.

This must serve to underline the necessity for research in trace mineral metabolism, an unexploited area of human physiology.

REFERENCES

(1) L.M. Klevay, "Elements of ischemic heart disease." *Perspectives in Biology and Medicine* 6, 186-192 (1977).

(2) K. Schwartz, "Essentiality versus toxicity of metals" in *Clinical Chemistry and Chemical Toxicology of Metals*. S. Brown ed. (Elsevier/North Holland, New York, 1977) 3-22.

(3) M. Anke et al, "Low nickel rations for growth and reproduction in pigs" in *Trace Element Metabolism in Animals* 2, J. Hoeckstra et al eds. (University Park Press, Baltimore, 1974) 715-718.

(4) H.A. Schroeder, "Municipal drinking water and cardiovascular death rates," *JAMA* 195, 81-85 (1966).

(5) J. Morris et al, "Hardness of local water supplies and mortality from cardiovascular disease," *Lancet* I, 860-862 (1962).

(6) T. Anderson et al, "Sudden death and ischemic heart disease," *New Engl. J. Med.* 280, 805-807 (1969).

(7) E. Bjorck et al, "On the relationship between water hardness and death rates in cardiovascular diseases," *Acta Med. Scand.* 239-262 (1965).

(8) K. Bresteker, "Hardness of drinking water and mortality, *T. Soc. Geneeska* 45, 658-660 (1967).

(9) T. Anderson et al, "Ischemic heart disease, water hardness and myocardial magnesium," *C.M.A.J.* 113, 199-204 (1975).

(10) R. Crawford and M.D. Crawford, "Prevalence and pathological changes of ischemic heart disease in a hard water and soft water area," *Lancet* I, 229-232 (1967).

(11) F.W. Stitt et al, "Clinical and biochemical indicators of cardiovascular disease among men living in hard and soft water areas," *Lancet* I, 122-126 (1973).

(12) T.R. Hartoma, "Serum zinc and copper and the geological environment in Finland," *Ann. Acad. Scient. Fenn. (Med.)* 171, 3-10 (1977).

(13) J. Kumpaleinen and R. Aaksaalii, "Chromium content of drinking water and cardiovascular disease," *Ann. Clin. Res.* 9, 79-86 (1977).

(14) T.P. Westermarck et al, "Selenium content of whole blood and serum in adults and children of different ages from different parts of Finland," *Acta Pharmacoll Toxicol.* 40, 465-475 (1977).

(15) R.L. McKenzie et al, "Selenium concentrations and glutathione peroxidase activity in blood of New Zealand infants and children," *Am. J. Clin. Nutr.* 31, 1413-1418 (1978).

(16) H.A. Schroeder et al, "Chromium deficiency as a factor in atherosclerosis," *J. Chron. Dis.* 23, 123-142 (1970).

(17) H.A. Schroeder et al, "Losses of vitamins and trace minerals from processing and preservation of foods," *Am. J. Clin. Nutr.* 24, 562-573 (1971).

(18) R.A. Levine et al, "Effects of oral chromium supplementation on the glucose tolerance of elderly human subjects," *Metab. Clin. Exp.* 17, 114-125 (1968).

(19) D. Kirkpatrick and D.E. Coffin, "The trace metal content of representative Canadian diets in 1970 and 1971," *J. Inst. Can Sci. Technol. Aliment* 7, 56-58 (1974).

(20) J.C. Meranger and D.C. Smith, "The heavy metal content of a typical Canadian diet," *Can. J. Public Health* 63, 53-57 (1972).

(21) A. Gormican, "Inorganic elements in foods used in hospital menus," *J. Am. Diet Assoc.* 56, 397-403 (1970).

(22) B.E. Guthrie, "Chromium, manganese, copper, zinc and cadmium content of New Zealand Foods," *N.Z.M.J.* 82, 418-424 (1975).

(23) E.W. Toepfer et al, "Chromium in foods in relation to biological activity, *J. Agr. Food Chem.* 21, 69-73 (1973).

(24) J.T. Kumpaleinen et al, "Urinary chromium excretion, *J. Agric. Food Chem.* 27, 490-494 (1979).

(25) L. Klevay, "Dietary copper and the copper requirements of man" in *Trace Elements −Metabolism in Man and Animals - 3.* M. Kirchgessner ed. (Institut fur Tiernahrungs Forschung, Freising, W. Germany, 1978) 307-311.

(26) J.M. Holden et al, "Zinc and copper in self-selected diets," *J. Am. Dietet. Assoc.* 75, 23-28 (1979).

(27) H. Spencer et al, "Metabolic balances of cadmium, copper, manganese and zinc in man," *Am. J. Clin. Nutr.* 32, 1867-1875 (1979).

(28) S.C. Vir et al, "Zinc and copper status of the elderly," *Am. J. Clin. Nutr.* 32, 1472-1476 (1979).

(29) W.H. Carnes, "Copper and connective tissue metabolism," *Int. Rev. Connect Tissue Res.* 4, 197-232 (1968).

(30) L. Klevay, "Hypercholesterolemia in rats produced by an increase in the ratio of zinc to copper," *Am. J. Clin. Nutr.* 26, 1060-1068 (1973).

(31) W.D. Caster and J.M. Doster, "Effect of the dietary zinc/copper ratio on plasma cholesterol level," *Nutr. Rep. Internat.* 19, 773-775 (1979).

(32) W. Woo and D.L. Gibbs, "Zinc and lipid metabolism," *Am. J. Clin. Nutr.* 33, 120-121 (1980).

(33) R.E. Shrader and G.J. Evenson, "Pancreatic pathology in manganese deficient guinea pigs," *J. Nutr.* 94, 269-281 (1968).

(34) R.M. Leach, "Role of manganese in mucopolysaccharide metabolism," *Fed. Proc.* 30, 991-994 (1971).

(35) K. Schwartz and W. Mertz, "Chromium (3) and the glucose tolerance factor," *Arch. Biochem. Biophys.* 85, 292-295 (1959).

(36) I.W.F. Davidson and W.L. Blackwel, "Changes in carbohydrate metabolism of squirrel monkeys with dietary chromium supplementation," *Proc. Soc. Exp. Med. Biol.* 127, 66-70 (1968).

(37) K. Schwartz and W. Mertz, "A physiological role for chromium(III) in glucose utilisation (glucose tolerance factor)," *Fed. Proc.* 20, 111-114 (1961).

(38) H.A. Schroeder, "Chromium deficiency in rats: A syndrome simulating growth," *J. Nutr.* 88, 439-445 (1965).

(39) W. Mertz et al, "Some aspects of glucose metabolism of chromium deficient rats raised in a strictly controlled environment," *J. Nutr.* 86, 107-112 (1965).

(40) H.A. Schroeder and J.J. Balassa, "Influence of chromium, cadmium and lead on rat aortic lipids and circulating cholesterol," *Am. J. Physiol.* 109, 433-437 (1965).

(41) H.A. Schroeder et al, "Effect of chromium, cadmium and lead on the growth and survival of rats," *J. Nutr.* 80, 48-54 (1963).

(42) N.J. Visek et al, "Metabolism of chromium 51 in animals as influenced by the chemical state," *Proc. Soc. Exp. Bioc. Med.* 41, 1349-1354 (1953).

(43) W. Mertz et al, "Effect of trivalent chromium complexes on glucose uptake by epididymal fat tissue of rats," *J. Biochem.* 236, 319-322 (1961).

(44) W. Mertz and D.E. Thurman, "Effects of yeast fractions on glucose metabolism of rat tissue in vitro," *Fed. Proc.* 27, 482-485 (1968).

(45) E.L. Tolman et al, "Effects of vanadium on glucose metabolism in vitro," *Life Sci.* 25, 1159-1164 (1969).

(46) H.E. Ganther et al, "Selenium and glutathione peroxidase–a review" in *Trace Elements in Human Health and Disease.* A Prasad ed. (Academic Press, New York, 1976) 165-234.

(47) K. Schwartz, "Role of vitamin E, selenium and related factors in experimental liver disease," *Fed. Proc.* 24, 58-67 (1965).

(48) E. Underwood, "Molybdenum" in *Trace Elements in Human and Animal Nutrition,* E.J. Underwood ed. (Academic Press, New York, 1977).

(49) K. Schwartz and S.C. Chen, "A bound form of silicon as a constituent of collagens," *Fed. Proc.* 33, 109-131 (1974).

(50) C.F. Mills, et al, "Mechanisms of the molybdenum:sulphur antagonism of copper utilisation by ruminants," *Op. cit.* (ref. 25) 150-159.

(51) C.H. Hill, "Chromium–Interactions with other metals," in *Chromium in Nutrition and Metabolism,* D. Shapcott and J. Hubert eds. (Elsevier, New York, 1980) 229-239.

(52) J. Versieck and R. Cornelis, "Normal levels of trace elements in human blood plasma or serum," *Anal. Chim. Acta.* 116, 217-254 (1980).

(53) F.H. Nielsen et al, "Evidence for a possible requirement of arsenic by the rat," *Fed. Proc.* 34, 923 (1975).

(54) A. Speecke et al, "Sampling of biological materials," *National Bureau of Standards Special Publication* 422 (1976).

(55) M. Barette (Personal Communication, 1980).

(56) J.A. Halsted et al, "A conspectus of research on zinc requirements in man," *J. Nutr.* 104, 345-397 (1974).

(57) S. Fells et al, "Urinary zinc levels as an indication of muscle catabolism," *Lancet* I, 280-282 (1973).

(58) K.M. Hambidge et al, "Low levels of zinc in hair, anorexia, poor growth and hypogeusia in children," *Pediatr. Res.* 6, 868-873 (1972).

(59) J.L. Greger and V.S. Sickles, "Saliva zinc levels: Potential indicators of zinc status," *Am. J. Nutr.* 32, 1859-1866 (1979).

(60) R.K. Berry et al, "Influence of dietary calcium, zinc and oil upon the in vitro uptake of zinc 65, by porcine red cells," *J. Nutr.* 88, 284 (1966).

(61) A.E. Harper, "Dietary goals: A skeptical view. 4th Arnold Beckman Conference," *Am. Assoc. for Clin. Chem.* (Oct., 1980).

(62) N.S.C. Chen et al, "Effect of chelating agents on chromium absorption in rats, *J. Nutr.* 103, 1182-1186 (1973).

(63) F.W. Sunderman et al, "Serum nickel after myocardial infarction," *New Eng. J. Med.* 283, 896-899 (1970).

(64) L.R. Nozdryukhina, "Use of blood trace elements for diagnosis of heart and liver disease," *Op. cit.* (ref. 25) 336-340.

(65) J.L. Taper et al, "Zinc and copper interaction and retention in elderly human subjects," *Fed. Proc.* 38, 430 (1978).

(66) C.S. Vir, "Zinc and copper status of the elderly," *Am. J. Clin. Nutr.* 32, 1472-1476 (1979).

(67) C.S. Vir, "Correction of impaired immunity in Down's syndrome by zinc," *Nutr. Rev.* 38, 365-367 (1980).

(68) A.S. Prasad et al, "Hypocupremia induced by zinc therapy in adults," *JAMA* 240, 2166-68 (1980).

(69) M. Abdulla, "Copper levels after oral zinc," *Lancet* I, 616 (1979).

(70) J.M. Morgan, "Hepatic chromium content in diabetic subjects," *Metab. Clin. Exptl.* 21, 313-316 (1972).

(71) D.J. Eatough et al, "Chromium in autopsy tissues of diabetic and non-diabetic American (Pima) Indians," *Op. cit.* (ref 25) 259-264.

(72) A.S. Abraham et al, "Serum chromium in patients with recent and old myocardial infarction," *Isr. heart, J.* 99, 604-606 (1980).

(73) H.A. Newman et al, "Serum chromium and angiographically determined coronary artery disease," *Clin. Chem.* 24, 541-544 (1978).

(74) D. Shapcott, "The detection of chromium deficiency," *Op. cit.* (ref. 51) 113-127.

(75) M.B. Rabinowitz et al, "Comparisons of chromium status in diabetic and normal men," *Metabolism* 29, 355-364 (1980).

(76) G. Saner in *Chromium in Nutrition and Disease* (Alan R. Liss Inc., New York, 1980).

(77) W. Canfield, "Chromium glucose tolerance and serum cholesterol in adults," *Op. cit.* (ref. 51), 145-161.

(78) G. Saner, "Chromium and glucose metabolism in children," *Op. cit.* (ref. 51), 129-145.

(79) R. Riales, "Influence of brewers' yeast on lipoprotein cholesterol," *Op. cit.* (ref. 51), 199-213.

(80) J.W. Rosson et al, "Hair chromium concentrations in adult insulin-treated diabetics," *Clin. Chim. Acta.* 93, 299-304 (1979).

(81) M.B. Rabinowitz et al, "Comparisons of chromium status in diabetic and normal men," *Metabolism* 29, 355-364 (1980).

(82) J.S. Vobecky et al, "Daily intake of chromium in infants," *Op. cit.* (ref. 51), 163-181.

(83) K.M. Hambidge and D. Rogerson, "Hair chromium levels in pregnant and non-pregnant women," *Am. J. Obstet. Gynecol.* 103, 320-324.

(84) D. Shapcott et al, "Hair chromium at delivery in relation to age and number of pregnancies," *Clin. Biochem.*, 129-131 (1980).

(85) K.M. Hambidge et al, "The concentration of chromium in the hair of normal children and children with juvenile diabetes mellitus," *Diabetes* 17, 515-519 (1968).

(86) J. Vobecky et al, "Hair and urine chromium content in 30 hospitalised female psychogeriatric patients and mentally healthy controls," *Nutr. Rep. Internat.* 22, 49-55 (1980).

(87) M. Anderson et al, "Chromium(III) trisacetylacetonate: an absorbable bioactive source of chromium," *Fed. Proc.* 40, 787 (1980).

-6-

Essential Fatty Acids and Chronic Degenerative Diseases

Hugh M. Sinclair

SUMMARY

In developed countries such as England and Wales, cardiovascular diseases account for about half the deaths in middle-aged men and cancer about a quarter. These and other "Western" chronic degenerative diseases have increased over the years and are today relatively rare in developing countries and in Japan. They were extremely rare in the vegetarian Hunzas and the carnivorous Eskimos on their traditional diets, and the latter diet is almost completely devoid of plant "fibre".

The Hunza and Eskimo diets are relatively very rich in essential fatty acids (EFA) and low in the antagonistic saturated fatty acids and *trans* isomers. There are two classes of EFA, linoleic and linolenic; these unsaturated fatty acids, like oleic which can be formed from carbohydrates, can be desaturated and elongated in the body. The functions of EFA are three: structural as part of the phosphoglycerides of cellular membranes, precursors of the prostanoids (prostaglandins, thromboxanes, prostacyclins, leukotrienes), and in the transport and oxidation of cholesterol. Although dietary EFA are predominantly in triglycerides, those in dietary phosphoglycerides are more active. The ratio in the tissues of the body of EFA to certain non-EFA that are antagonistic (long-chain saturated fatty acids and *trans* isomers) is the important factor in determining susceptibility to chronic degenerative diseases.

The possible relation of faulty cellular membranes, arising from a relative deficiency of EFA, to chronic degenerative diseases is discussed, particularly in relation to Japanese and Eskimos.

CHRONIC DEGENERATIVE DISEASES

Mortality from different diseases varies greatly between different countries, but in general the greatest variation is between the developed and developing countries. In the latter protein-energy malnutrition and kwashiorkor are prevalent amongst infants and young children, whereas in most developed countries ischaemic heart disease (IHD) is a major cause of death in adults. This chapter will be concerned with killer diseases in the developed countries, and only for these are good mortality statistics available. Amongst them the main causes of death vary.

The expectation of life of a man aged 45 in 1974/5 was highest in the following six countries of the 40 listed by WHO:[1] Greece (31.7 years), Costa Rica (31.5), Cuba (31.3), Iceland (31.1), Sweden (30.2), Japan (30.1); it was lowest in Mauritius (24.5), Finland (25.9), Chile (26.2), Czechoslovakia (26.3), Northern Ireland (26.3), Scotland (26.5). Ischaemic heart disease (A83) accounted for the following deaths per 100,000 population in males aged 45-54 in 1974: Thailand 5.2, Japan 30.4, Scotland 364.9. Malignant neoplasms are in general rare in developing countries; and most forms are much rarer in Japan than in other developed countries, gastric carcinoma being a notable exception. Age-adjusted male death rates for certain forms in Scotland and Japan in 1975 were:[2] for lung (A51), Scotland 84.8, Japan 19.9; for colon (A48), Scotland 15.4, Japan 5.1; for stomach (A47), Scotland 19.9, Japan 55.9; and for breast in women (A54), Scotland 25.8, Japan 5.0.

The most interesting fact in clinical medicine is that the expectation of life of a middle-aged man in developed countries in the last century has hardly altered. In England and Wales for a man aged 50 years it was 20.02 years in 1841 and 22.7 in 1975. Yet 1841 was before almost every great medical advance: anaesthesia, antiseptic surgery, antibiotics, hormones, drugs used today except derivatives of opium, modern sanitation. In 1841 William Farr believed most such middle-aged men died of tuberculosis and acute lobar pneumonia, causes of death that are today rare amongst them; but then few deaths were attributed to the chronic degenerative diseases such as IHD and cancer which are such common killing diseases today. If such diseases have increased rapidly in developed countries there must be a cause and as a student in the 1930s I thought the cause must be nutritional and the dietary change an alteration in essential fatty acids (EFA) or possibly in trace elements as we increasingly processed and sophisticated foods. A hint is given by an alteration in the rise in mortality (allowing for changes in classification) when a national dietary change occurs. In European countries for which figures are available deaths attributed to IHD were increasing up to 1939 but then levelled or even fell throughout the War; in England and Wales however they started to rise again in 1943 and a change in diet occurred in 1942 with Lend-Lease causing an increase in saturated fat from margarine, fat bacon and a curious food called "spam". As will be discussed below, free saturated fatty acids cause an immediate alteration in the thrombotic tendency of blood and the rapidity with which the nation's mortality from IHD followed this change in diet must be caused by this (if indeed the two are related) rather than by an alteration in atherosclerosis which is a chronic process.

There have been other alterations in the rise in IHD. In England and Wales a report in 1978 of the Government Statistical Service[3] called attention to the striking increase in mortality due to circulatory diseases particularly IHD in middle-aged men over the last 40 years and suggested that the falling trends in 1971-5 might be due to mild winters and the absence of a severe influenza epidemic. In the U.S. there has been a dramatic fall in deaths from IHD since 1968. Various risk factors have diminished: since 1966 the number of male cigarette-smokers has decreased by 25 percent, in 1972 the High Blood Pressure Education Program was introduced, and in 1978 Levy further stated[4] that "Between 1963 and 1975, there has been a 56.7% decline in the consumption of animal fats and oils, a 19.2% decline in the consumption of fluid milk and cream, a 31.9% decline in butter consumption, and a 12.6% decline in egg consumption. In the past 10 years, a 4.8% decrease in plasma cholesterol levels in the United States has been reported".

We may summarise certain present killer diseases in men aged 45-54 years in England and Wales in 1978 as follows.[5] All circulatory disorders (ICD 390-458) accounted for 52% of all deaths, with IHD (ICD 410-414) accounting for 41% of all. Neoplasms (ICD 140-239) caused 27% of all deaths, respiratory diseases (ICD 460-519) 5.8%, accidents with poisoning and violence 7.2%. Neoplasms of particular sites accounted for the following percentages of deaths from all neoplasms: lung (ICD 162/3) 38.3, stomach (ICD 151) 8.4, colon (ICD 153) 6.2, bladder (ICD 188) 2.3, prostate (ICD 185) 1.1.

HYPOTHESES RELATING DIET TO KILLER DISEASES

As various authors in this book are putting forward various hypotheses, only brief comments will be given here about them. The vegetarian Hunzas and the carnivorous Eskimos are two very different populations in which the "Western" chronic degenerative diseases were very rare. Sir Robert McCarrison lived as the only medical officer for seven years amongst the 10,000 Hunzas high in the Himalayas. He found they lived to a great age, had superb physique, and remarkable agility and endurance. He saw no case of heart disease, cancer, appendicitis, peptic ulcer, mucous colitis, multiple sclerosis or diabetes mellitus. Their diet was mainly whole grains (wheat, barley and maize), vegetables and fruits especially sun-dried apricots; some milk and butter were eaten but meat only at feasts, and no alcohol. This diet is relatively high in linoleic and linolenic acids and low in saturated fat, also extremely high in carotenoids since dried apricots are a very rich source (and rich in iron), and high in ascorbic acid. "When the severe nature of the winter in that part of the Himalayas is considered, and the fact that their housing accommodation and conservancy arrangements are of the most primitive, it becomes obvious that the enforced restriction to the unsophisticated foodstuffs of nature is compatible with long life, continued vigour, and perfect physique".[6]

This almost completely vegetarian diet is very rich in fibre. McCarrison[6] was impressed with the importance of indigestible material in the diet. "In addition to proteins, carbohydrates, fats, mineral salts and vitamins, there are in food blood-forming substances, extractives, flavouring matter and pigments that have parts of greater or lesser importance to play in the nourishment of the body. The food must also contain a certain amount of innocuous, indigestible material, or roughage as it is called, to stimulate intestinal movements". Others had also stressed the importance of roughage or bran or fibre as is mentioned in the introduction to the recent comprehensive report on *Medical*

Aspects of Dietary Fibre by a Working Party of the Royal College of Physicians of London.[7] This, although surprisingly being unable to conclude that brown bread has greater merit than white in terms of health and better nutrition, follows convention in considering dietary fibre as being solely of plant origin: "Dietary fibre is a convenient term for the supporting structures of plant cell walls and the substances intimately associated with them". Trowell and others in 1976 wrote[7] that "dietary fibre should be redefined . . . as the plant polysaccharides and lignin which are resistant to hydrolysis by the digestive enzymes of man". I pointed out in 1978 that the word 'plant' should be omitted from such definitions since there is no good reason for excluding unabsorbed animal mucopolysaccharides.[8] This is especially important in relation to strict carnivores such as Eskimos who have none of the diseases attributed by Cleave, Burkitt, Trowell and others to lack of dietary fibre: IHD, cancer of colon and breast, diabetes mellitus, appendicitis, gall-stones, diverticular disease, ulcerative colitis and Crohn's disease, hiatus hernia, varicose veins, haemorrhoids, dental caries.[7] But Eskimos have bulky faeces from unabsorbed residues of collagen and mucopolysaccharides; they eat skin and tendons of animals they catch. Some long-chain fatty acids are unabsorbed and we found on students that timnodonic (C20:5) and clupanodonic (C22:6) acids if eaten in large amounts decreased transit time and appeared in faeces. The Eskimos Drs. Bang and Dyerberg and I studied in N.W. Greenland in 1976, who were partially on "Western" foods,[9] all excreted in the faeces small amounts of gadoleic (C20:1) and cetoleic acids (C22:1); on an Eskimo diet of seal and fish[10] I also excreted these as well as small amounts of C20:5 and C22:6. I believe that instead of plant fibre we should in the context of "roughage" consider all the unabsorbed residue of foods, whether carbohydrate (such as most plant fibre), protein (such as collagen), fat (such as long-chain fatty acids and plant sterols), and inorganic compounds or the salts of unabsorbed organic compounds (such as calcium and zinc phytates).

I first met McCarrison when I was a student intending to study nutrition and learned from him about the Hunzas. As soon as I qualified in medicine in 1937 I went to the U.S. to see the work being done on rats on the recently discovered EFA. I wanted to study Eskimos because they had the highest dietary fat of any race, but very rich in polyunsaturated fats characteristic of Arctic plants and animals. In March 1943 I had the opportunity, when undertaking some Wartime work at the request of the Royal Canadian Air Force, of examining Canadian Indians and Eskimos in the Canadian Arctic; the expedition was jointly sponsored by the RCAF and the Canadian Government. I was particularly interested in the alleged extreme rarity amongst them of chronic degenerative diseases such as heart disease and cancer, although clearly statistics were unreliable, and infections and accidents caused the expectation of life to be low; subsequently I had the advantage of several discussions with Stefansson, the greatest authority on Eskimos. Since during this wartime visit no biochemical estimations could be made, I used a slit-lamp microscope with crossed polaroids to examine their eyes for deposition of cholesterol (arcus senilis and cataract) and found none even in old subjects (ages unfortunately unascertainable); but examination of young British and New Zealand pilots (average age 23 years) being trained at the same latitude showed that 10% (number examined 131) had some degree of arcus senilis. Arcus senilis does not necessarily indicate the presence of atheroma, but the latter if severe is usually accompanied by arcus as in Type II hyperlipoproteinaemia. The diet of true Eskimos (eating fish, seal, whale, some caribou and occasional berries in summer but with some "Western" foods from trappers) was estimated to provide about 3,360 kcal from 377 g of protein (all animal protein), 59 g of carbohydrate and 162 g of fat.[11] This is more than five times as much protein and 1½ times as much fat as we consume. But the fat is quite different in quality to ours, being extremely rich in polyunsaturated fatty acids of the linolenic class (n-3), which are characteristic of fish. I have always maintained,[12] despite opposition twenty years ago from Thomasson[13] and Ahrens[14] and Holman,[15] that the linolenic as well as the linoleic class are essential fatty acids; C22:6w3 is it appears an obligatory fatty acid of the nervous system and after birth must be derived from a dietary fatty acid of the linolenic class. If series-3 prostaglandins are essential, they must be derived from fatty acids of this class of EFA. It was mainly because of this very high animal fat diet (but very high in EFA) that I was and am particularly interested in studying Eskimos and further recent work will be discussed below after considering the nature and function of EFA.

ESSENTIAL FATTY ACIDS

EFA are not synonymous with polyunsaturated fatty acids. We are concerned with three classes of fatty acids: EFA, certain non-EFA that are antagonistic to them and include long-chain saturated fatty acids and *trans* isomers of EFA, and certain monounsaturated fatty acids. Fatty acids are conveniently written by placing the number of carbon atoms after C, the number of *cis* double bonds after a colon, and the position of the first double bond from the methyl end after n- assuming all other double bonds to be methylene-interrupted. Thus, linoleic acid is C18:2n-6 or $CH_3(CH_2)_4CH=CHCH_2CH=CH(CH_2)_7COOH$. The body can desaturate and elongate fatty acids thereby converting linoleic to arachidonic (C20:4n-6), linolenic (C18:3n-3) to timnodonic (C20:5n-3) and clupanodonic (C22:6n-3), and oleic (C18:1n-9) to eicosatrienoic (C20:3n-9). But it cannot convert one class into another (e.g., n-6 to n-3), cannot make linoleic or linolenic, but can make oleic and therefore the polyunsaturated fatty acid C20:3n-9 from saturated fatty acids or carbohydrate. The oleic class (n-9) and the less prevalent palmitoleic (C16:1n-7) class of monounsaturated fatty acids are neutral in the context of discussing EFA being neither essential nor antagonistic. But two monounsaturated fatty acids, erucic (C22:1n-9) and cetoleic (C22:1n-11), are very important in that they are toxic[16] and in consequence there are for erucic EEC regulations (accepted by the British Government) limiting the amount allowed in foods to 5%. It is therefore surprising that the most recent Report of the Food Standards Committee of the British Ministry of Agriculture, Fisheries and Food states[17] that "mono-unsaturated fatty acids . . . would seem to have no special function in the diet". Cetoleic acid will be mentioned again later. Fatty acids relevant to EFA can be summarised in a diagram from an earlier paper.[18]

Fatty acids
- EFA
  - Linoleic (C18 : 2n-6) . . . . . > Arachidonic (C20 : 4n-6)
  - Linolenic (C18 : 3n-3) . . . . . > Timnodonic (C20 : 5n-3)
- Non-EFA
  - Not antagonistic: Oleic (C18 : 1n-9) . . . . . > Eicosapentaenoic (C20 : 3n-9)
  - Antagonistic:
    - Isomers of EFA, e.g. { trans-linoleic Elaeostearic }
    - Long-chain saturated, e.g. { Palmitic (C16 : 0) Stearic (C18 : 0) }

Polyunsaturated

Saturated

EFA are more prevalent in plant than animal foods in "Western" diets. Linoleic acid is found abundantly in many vegetable seed oils (e.g., safflower, corn, sunflower, soyabean) and linolenic acid is the most common fatty acid of leaves such as grass (which however have little total fat). But ruminant animals (i.e., cattle, sheep) have little EFA in their adipose tissue and milk or butter since the microflora in the rumen destroy the linolenic acid in the fodder and make more saturated fatty acids and isomers.

Most fatty acids in foods are contained in the triglycerides found in adipose tissue, between muscle fibres in meats and in vegetable seed oils, butter, margarine, cooking fats and milk. Cellular membranes, however, are rich in phosphoglycerides which contain a high proportion of polyunsaturated fatty acids—linoleic and arachidonic acids in those of land animals and timnodonic in the phosphoglycerides of marine animals. Liver is a particularly rich source. The composition of adipose tissue reflects the diet of the animal: pigs in Britain tended to be free-ranging and had "soft" (unsaturated) body fat until 1939, when a change in husbandry and in marketing caused them to be fed to produce "hard" (saturated) fat.

Although quantitatively the fatty acids in dietary phosphoglycerides are much less than those in triglycerides, the former have an advantage that has not been considered in dietary calculations. In 1947 we found that linoleic acid fed to EFA-deficient rats in a phosphoglyceride (lecithin) was much more effective in curing the deficiency than if fed as a triglyceride or ethyl ester. Unfortunately the "lecithin" available then was highly impure and we did not investigate this further. In 1956 Mead and colleagues[19] showed that EFA-deficient mice fed labelled methyl linoleate oxidised it faster to respiratory CO_2 than did normal mice and it was not obvious why if this EFA was so rapidly wasted animals were not easily deficient. I suggested that since phosphoglycerides were not used for energy, they should be more effective since they were directly available for the main function of EFA—incorporation as phosphoglycerides into cellular membranes.

Ingested phosphoglycerides are mainly hydrolysed in the small intestine by pancreatic phospholipase A_2 which removes the fatty acid from the 2-position;

this fatty acid is usually an EFA. Within the mucosal cells re-esterification occurs preferentially with EFA from the lipid pool in the cells. Detailed work by the German firm of Nattermann[20],[21] has shown in rats that on feeding lecithin with both fatty acids and choline labelled with ^{3}H and ^{14}C, some 75% of the label appears in the triglycerides of chylomicrons in thoracic lymph, 25% in the resynthesised lecithin, and possibly a small amount of lecithin is absorbed unchanged. Obviously a greater amount of EFA will be found in the phosphoglycerides of chylomicrons if there is an EFA in the 1-position (which occurs when occasionally both acyl groups are EFA) or when the mucosal pool is rich in EFA so that the preferential reacylation of the absorbed lyso-compound with EFA occurs as is achieved by also ingesting triglyceride rich in EFA.

A recent study in man has shown[22] that when lecithin and safflower oil supplied equal amounts of oral fatty acids, in contrast with the rat more were found in the triglyceride of chylomicrons from safflower oil than from lecithin; intestinal infusion of lecithin produced small chylomicrons or VLDL with a higher ratio of coat-to-core lipids than is obtained with larger chylomicrons after infusion of triglycerides. The authors point out that, in accordance with the views of Tall and Small[23] that the surface components (phosphoglycerides, cholesterol and apoproteins) of chylomicrons can contribute to the formation of HDL, the small chylomicrons from dietary phosphoglycerides might be beneficial in this respect. In a paper to the ISF/AOCS World Congress in May 1980, Houtsmuller[24] stated that the chylomicron lecithin was transferred particularly to HDL, and linoleic acid in lecithin was somewhat more active in curing EFA-deficient rats than in a triglyceride. So the form in which EFA are included in the diet should be considered.

The functions of EFA are three. First, as just mentioned they are constituents of the phosphoglycerides of cellular membranes. Secondly, they are concerned in the transport and hepatic oxidation of cholesterol, cholesteryl linoleate being the predominant ester in plasma. Adams[25] found that the relative sclerogenic properties of cholesterol and its esters ranked in decreasing order: monosaturated, free, saturated, C18:2, C18:3, C20:4. But when he[26] implanted free and esterified cholesterol subcutaneously in rats, the resorption was slower than free cholesterol in the case of saturated and monoene and diene esters, but more rapid in the case of triene and tetraene esters. By analogy, the pentaene and hexaene esters formed from dietary fatty acids of marine oils would be even more rapidly transported.

The third function of EFA is in the formation of prostanoids, such as prostaglandins, thromboxanes, prostacyclins and leukotrienes. The relationship of these to thrombosis and ischaemic heart disease has recently been discussed by me elsewhere,[18] and an excellent account is given by Jorgensen and Dyerberg.[27] In brief summary, the EFA C20:4 gives rise to a prostaglandin, PGD2, that disaggregates platelets and in vessel walls to a prostacyclin, PGI2, that Vane and his colleagues[28] showed to be the most active known disaggregating compound; platelets however convert C20:4 to a thromboxane, TXA2, that aggregates them. The EFA C20:5 from marine oils gives rise to a disaggregating prostaglandin PGD3 which is inhibited by PGE2 but not by PGE3;[29] vessel walls form from C20:5 a strongly disaggregating PGI3[30] and platelets a thromboxane TXA3 that does not affect them. So C20:5 is disaggregating which explains the lack of thrombotic complications[31] and well known prolonged bleeding time[32] of Eskimos, and the very long bleeding time and spontaneous haemorrhages that I had on an Eskimo diet.[10]

A further function of EFA, perhaps mainly but not entirely through prostanoids, is their role in immune reactions, reviewed by Meade and Mertin.[33]

Important though EFA are in forming prostanoids, there is no doubt that the structural function in cellular membranes is the most important. For instance, Unilever Research in Vlaardingen have made the important discovery[34] that in the rat columbinic acid (which is linoleic acid with an extra *trans* double bond) will prevent or cure the lesions of deficiency of EFA (except those of the kidney) but does not give rise to prostanoids. The fluidity of cellular membranes is largely determined by the fatty acids in the phosphoglycerides, all-*cis* polyunsaturated fatty acids increasing this. Further, at each *cis* double bond the fatty-acid chain is kinked, so that arachidonic acid with four such bonds is in the form of a U. It is suggested[35] that the free cholesterol in cellular membranes is fitted into the curve of the EFA in the 2-position of the phosphoglyceride. Clearly with saturated fatty acids or *trans* isomers, both of which have straight chains, faulty membranes will be formed, and this occurs in a relative deficiency of EFA, which means a low ratio of EFA to such non-EFA at the site where new cellular membranes are being formed.

POSSIBLE RELATION OF A RELATIVE DEFICIENCY OF EFA TO CHRONIC DEGENERATIVE DISEASES

It is obvious therefore that this relative deficiency, caused for instance by a high dietary ratio of saturated fat to EFA or of excess sugar which gives rise in the body to saturated fat, will cause faulty membranes that can make tissues unusually permeable and also susceptible to a variety of insults such as ultraviolet light, x-rays, infections, carcinogens, toxic substances. Since the requirement of EFA is about seven times greater in male lower animals than in female during the period of reproductive activity, lesions attributable to a relative deficiency of EFA might be expected to be more common in men than women until the menopause.

I have mentioned above that I have been interested since a student in this relative deficiency of EFA in "Western" diets being mainly responsible for the chronic degenerative "Western" diseases, and for the rise of these to the increasing relative deficiency as we process and sophisticate foods more and more to give foods a greater shelf-life, and feed animals to produce saturated fat.[36] As already mentioned such diseases are very rare in such different peoples on their traditional diets as vegetarian Hunzas, carnivorous Eskimos and omnivorous Japanese, but are appearing now that these diets are becoming "Westernised". Stefansson[37] in his last book, of which I read the proofs for him, marshalled the evidence that cancer (except for certain special forms such as carcinoma of stomach in Japanese and of liver in Africans from aflatoxin) is relatively very rare in developing countries; it was almost unknown even in long-lived Eskimos despite their traditional diet being the highest in fat of any people, but this fat is relatively very rich in the long-chain EFA of the linolenic class.

Many authors, for instance Armstrong and Doll,[38] have correlated high dietary fat with carcinoma of colon, rectum, breast, ovary, prostate and endometrium; but the absence in Eskimos does not support this. The Japanese diet is low in total fat but relatively rich in EFA (from C20:5 and C22:6 in marine food, C18:2 in soyabean oil and C18:3 in this and in vegetables); despite a high consumption of cigarettes, age-adjusted deaths from cancer of the trachea, bronchus and lung (A51) in 1975 was only 19.86 in Japan as compared with 84.76 in Scotland.[2] It is possible that a relative deficiency of EFA could make the epithelial cells more susceptible to a chemical carcinogen in cigarette-smoke which could also account for the unusually high incidence in different countries in males (allowing for differences in smoking) and the greatly increasing incidence of deaths over the years which outstrips the increase in smoking (allowing for a 20-year or so lag between number of cigarettes smoked and mortality).

I have mentioned above that Eskimos were in general short-lived because of the high prevalence of accidents and to a lesser extent infections. Japanese and Hunzas however were not. Since about 1950 Eskimos have received considerable amounts of "Western" foods including sugar and white flour; their diseases have in consequence altered. For 30 years some statistics showing these diseases have become available; for instance on 27 May 1950 the Act on Health Services in Greenland was passed and an annual report is issued by the Chief Medical Officer. According to official figures, the percentage age-distribution on 1 July 1975 of persons born and living in Greeland[39] (not all of whom were Eskimos) as compared with that for England and Wales in 1972[40] was as follows:

Percentage Age Distribution

	0–14	15–19	20–24	25–29	30–34	35–39	40–44
Greenland	41.9	11.4	8.4	6.2	6.4	5.2	5.0
England and Wales	23.8	7.0	7.3	7.2	5.9	5.7	5.9

	45–49	50–54	55–59	60–64	65–69	70–74	75+
Greenland	4.4	2.8	2.5	2.0	1.6	1.1	0.85
England and Wales	6.2	6.2	5.9	5.9	4.9	3.7	4.6

The following are deaths per 100,000 population, all ages, for males in England and Wales in 1978 and both sexes in Greenland in 1971:

Deaths per 100,000 Population

Cause	(ICD)	England and Wales	Greenland
All	—	1,236	544
Cancer	(140–239)	287	67
IHD	(410–414)	386	52
Vascular disorders of nervous system	(430–438)	117	29
Pneumonia	(480–486)	91	58
Bronchitis	(490–493)	72	33
Accidents*	—	34	140

*In England and Wales including 19 from motor vehicles.

In the Umanak district of N.W. Greenland the population on 1 January 1974 was 2,652 of whom 2,246 were born in Greenland. In Umanak Hospital (33 beds including children) in the 11 years 1964 to 1974 the following numbers of patients were admitted: IHD, 18; cerebrovascular disease, 6 (in 1973 and 1974); varicose veins, 3; hypertensive heart disease, 0; cancer of stomach, 3 (all in 1974); of intestine including rectum, 1; of lung, 6 (in 1973 and 1974); of breast, 0; bronchitis, 92; tuberculosis, 105; cholecystitis, 14; ulcerative colitis, Crohn's disease, diverticulitis, 5 (in 1973 and 1974); rheumatoid arthritis, 22; prolapsed disc, 10; fracture of neck of femur, 12 (8 in 1972-4); multiple sclerosis, 0; diabetes mellitus, 2. During these years many of these diseases appeared which were rare before, especially IHD and cancer; two gastrointestinal disorders, previously very rare, became fairly common, the admissions for peptic ulcers being 35 and for appendicitis 67 in the eleven years. There are occasional crises: in December 1959 400 persons in Umanak had severe gastroenteritis from eating a dead dolphin.

It is not possible here to review the evidence for the rarity amongst Eskimos when on their traditional diet of the "Western" chronic degenerative diseases, or for the rise in these during the past thirty years when the diet has been dramatically changed. Absence of good figures for mortality and morbidity, of autopsies and even of age make assessment difficult; as mentioned above, the Canadian Eskimos I examined in 1943, who had for years had some access to "Western" foods, were short-lived mainly through accidents and usually did not know their ages; longevity was discussed by Stefansson[41] and Rousselière.[42] Reference to some of the literature, particularly the extensive publications of Bertelsen[43] and the early work of Rabinowitch[44] was made elsewhere.[11] Scott, who published serum cholesterol levels of Alaskan Eskimo men,[45] had pointed out that in 1955 probably no Eskimos in Alaska subsisted on wholly native diets and figures he published for purchases from stores in 1945-49 showed the extensive use of flour, sugar, saturated fats and other "Western" foods.[46] Schaefer[47] has written extensively in recent years on the Canadian Eskimos and there have been recent studies of Alaskan Eskimos, including autopsies[48] and plasma cholesterol values,[49,50] but these people are not on their traditional diet and only these studies and those of Bang and his colleagues[51] in Umanak were considered by McGill[52] who concluded that their serum cholesterol values were high.

The tendency to bleed in Eskimos,[32] and the dramatic increase in bleeding-time I experienced when on an Eskimo diet,[10] are partly explained by the prevalence of C20:5 rather than C20:4 in their diet and body as discussed above. But I believe an alteration in the structure of platelet membranes is also responsible since on an Eskimo diet my bleeding-time was very much more prolonged than was possible by inhibiting with aspirin the cyclo-oxygenase that makes prostanoids.

Several of the diseases mentioned above which have been appearing amongst Eskimos since "Western" foods became easily available have also been increasing in developed countries; for instance Elliot-Smith[53] called attention to the rise in Oxford of acute appendicitis, a disease rare at the beginning of the century. At the same symposium ten years ago I briefly tried to explain[54] how a relative deficience of EFA might contribute to this and other diseases that were increasing but Elliot-Smith preferred the conclusion of Cleave, who also contributed to the symposium,[55] that excess of sugar and refining of flour is responsible for the rise of these killer diseases.[56] Elsewhere I have discussed the importance of the refining of flour.[57] Excess sugar, as mentioned above, leads to saturated fat in the body and hence to a relative deficiency of EFA unless EFA are also included; at the cellular level it does not matter whether the saturated fat comes from dietary fat or sugar. Elliot-Smith stated:[53] "Animal fat has been blamed for a lot of present diseases, but it is an extraordinary thing that a substance which man has been consuming for thousands of years should suddenly in the 20th century become poisonous to him!" But "animal fat" can be rich in EFA, as in fatty fish, or very poor as in stall-fed cattle; it can in a particular animal, such as pigs or poultry, be rich or poor according to how the animal is fed.

The structural function of EFA in cellular membranes and connective tissue could contribute to the rise in developed countries and the rarity in under-developed of certain gastrointestinal disorders, for instance by increasing the liability to infection and hence acute appendicitis, or to the absorption of substances giving rise to allergy that might be important in ulcerative colitis, or to solid particles that are absorbed into the lymphatics and might cause Crohn's disease, or to increased susceptibility to intraluminal pressure that might cause diverticulosis. The structural relation of EFA to multiple sclerosis has recently been summarised elsewhere[58] and in the same place Swank[59] summarised his work on the relation of total dietary fat to this disease. A dramatic change occurs in connective tissue such as the cartilage of the ear in lower animals deficient in EFA;[60] a relative deficiency in man might contribute to senile osteoporosis and prolapsed discs. Rheumatoid arthritis was extremely rare in Eskimos but is now becoming prevalent as figures given above for Umanak show; cod-liver oil has been claimed particularly by Russian workers to be useful in treatment. Articular cartilage contains a third of its lipid as glycerophosphatides and about 15% of the total fatty acids are EFA.[61]

Various studies[62,63] have shown that diabetes mellitus is almost unknown amongst Eskimos on their traditional diet. As discussed previously[64] the structural function of EFA could account for the diabetic triopathy. The diabetic, with increased requirement of EFA, has increased capillary fragility as has the lower animal deficient in EFA, and chronic deficiency might deplete peripheral nerves of EFA and cause the neuropathy. Houtsmuller and his colleagues[65] have shown in a controlled trial that a diet high in linoleic acid resulted in significantly less retinopathy and electrocardiographic abnormalities. In lower animals the contractility and perfusion rate of the heart are improved.[66] This is only one of the advantageous cardiovascular effects of EFA, others being the decrease in LDL and VLDL, the increase in HDL, the markedly decreased thrombogenic tendency of platelets, and the demonstration by Iacono and his colleagues[67] that a diet high in EFA reduces blood-pressure in man, just as it reduces salt-induced hypertension in lower animals.[68] But the high amount of long-chain EFA from fish in the Japanese diet does not overcome the prevalent hypertension. Experiments carried out by Unilever Research[66] show that the effect of linoleic acid on salt-induced hypertension in rats is probably exerted through prostaglandins. In pre-eclamptic toxaemia, usually arising after the twenty-fourth week of pregnancy, there is an increase in the customary greater thrombotic tendency of blood characteristic of late pregnancy, with hypertension, oedema, proteinuria, retinopathy and other clinical signs. Pre-eclampsia does not seem to occur in Eskimos on their traditional diet; it may be related to a relative deficiency of prostacyclin as suggested by Lewis and colleagues[69] who found that increased amounts are produced normally in late pregnancy.

Two other conditions almost unknown in Eskimos on their traditional diet are acne vulgaris and dental caries, but both are now prevalent. The degree of dental caries in the children of the Umanak district where the consumption of sugar is now very high[9] is much worse than even in British children of the same age; but these are not killer diseases.

Much more research is urgently needed to define the possible relation of a relative deficiency of essential fatty acids to the chronic degenerative diseases that are increasingly prevalent in those developed countries in which this deficiency occurs and are rare in those countries where the diet is relatively rich in EFA of either class whether the diet is very high in total fat as in the Eskimo or low as in the Japanese. We should plan to reduce long-chain saturated fatty acids and *trans* isomers in the diet and increase EFA of both classes by including certain vegetable seed oils, polyunsaturated margarines, offal and fish such as mackerel.

REFERENCES

(1) World Health Organisation, *World Health Statistics Annual* 1 (WHO, Geneva, 1977).
(2) M. Segi, "Age-adjusted death rates for cancer for selected sites (A-classification) in 46 countries in 1975" (Japan, Nagoya, 1980).
(3) Office of Population Censuses and Surveys, Ser. DH1 no. 3 (HMSO, London, 1978).
(4) R. Levy, "Progress in prevention of cardiovascular disease," *Prev. Med.* 7, 464-475 (1978).
(5) Office of Population Censuses and Surveys. Ser. DH2 no. 5 (HMSO, London, 1978).
(6) Sir R. McCarrison and H.M. Sinclair, *Nutrition and Health* (Faber and Faber, London, 1961).

(7) Royal College of Physicians of London, *Medical Aspects of Dietary Fibre* (Pitman Medical, London, 1980).

(8) H.M. Sinclair, "The human nutritional advantages of plant foods over animal foods," *Qual. Plant Pl. Fds human Nutr.* 29, 7-18 (1979).

(9) H.O. Bang, J. Dyerberg and H.M. Sinclair, "The Diet of Greenland Eskimos," *Amer. J. clin. Nutr.* 9 (In press).

(10) H.M. Sinclair, "Advantages and disadvantages of an Eskimo diet," *Drugs Affecting Lipid Metabolism*, R. Fumagalli, D. Kritchevsky and R. Paoletti (eds.) (Elsevier, Amsterdam, 1980) 363-370.

(11) H.M. Sinclair, "The diet of Canadian Indians and Eskimos," *Proc. Nutr. Soc.* 12, 69-82 (1953).

(12) H.M. Sinclair, "Supply and dietary use of fats," *Lancet* I, 474-475 (1959).

(13) H.J. Thomasson, "Biological standardization of essential fatty acids (a new method)," *Internat. Rev. Vitamin Res.* 25, 62-82 (1953).

(14) E.H. Ahrens Jr., W. Insull Jr., J. Hirsch, W. Stoffel, M.L. Peterson, J.W. Farquhar, T. Miller and H.J. Thomasson, "The effect on human serum-lipids of a dietary fat, highly unsaturated, but poor in essential fatty acids," *Lancet* I, 115-119 (1959).

(15) R.T. Holman, "Biological activities of and requirements for polyunsaturated acids," *Prog. Chem. Fats other lipids* 9, 607-682 (1969).

(16) J.L. Beare-Rogers, "Docosenoic acids in dietary fats," *Prog. Chem. Fats other lipids* 15, 29-56 (1977).

(17) Ministry of Agriculture, Fisheries and Food, "Food Standards Committee, Second Report, On Claims and Misleading Descriptions" (HMSO, London, 1980).

(18) H.M. Sinclair, "Prevention of coronary heart disease: the role of essential fatty acids," *Postgrad. med. J.* 56, 579-584 (1980).

(19) J.F. Mead, W.H. Slaton and A.B. Decker, "Metabolism of the essential fatty acids. II. The metabolism of stearate, oleate, and linoleate by fat-deficient and normal mice," *J. biol. Chem.* 218, 401-407 (1956).

(20) D. Le Kim and H. Betzing, "Intestinal absorption of polyunsaturated phosphatidyl-choline in the rat," *Hoppe-Seyler's Z. Physiol. Chem.* 357, 1321-1331 (1976).

(21) D. Lekim, "On the pharmacokinetics of orally applied Essential Phospholipids (EPL)." In "Phosphatidyl-choline," H. Peeters (ed.) (Springer-Verlag, Berlin, 1976) 48-65.

(22) F.U. Beil and S.M. Grundy, "Studies on plasma lipoproteins during absorption of exogenous lecithin in man," *J. Lipid Res.* 21, 525-536 (1980).

(23) A.R. Tall and D.M. Small, "Body cholesterol removal: role of plasma high-density lipoproteins," *Adv. Lipid Res.* 17, 2-51 (1980).

(24) U.M.T. Houtsmuller, "Metabolic fate of dietary lecithin," *ISF/AOCS World Congress*, abs. 159 (1980).

(25) Y.H. Abdulla, C.W.M. Adams and R.S. Morgan, "Connective-tissue reactions to implantation of purified sterol, sterol esters, phosphoglycerides, glycerides and free fatty acids," *J. Path. Bact.* 94, 63 (1967).

(26) Y.H. Abdulla, C.W.M. Adams and R.S. Morgan, "Differential resorption rates of subcutaneous implants of ^{3}H cholesterol, various ^{3}H cholesterol esters and ^{3}H cholesterol 1-^{14}C linolenate." *J. Atheroscler. Res.* 9, 81-85 (1969).

(27) K.A. Jorgensen and J. Dyerberg, "Platelets and atherosclerosis," *Danish med. Bull.* 27, 253-260 (1980).

(28) S. Moncada, R. Gryglewski, S. Bunting and J.R. Vane, "An enzyme isolated from arteries transforms prostaglandin endoperoxides to an unstable substance that inhibits platelet aggregation," *Nature* 263, 663-665 (1976).

(29) R.J. Gryglewski, J.A. Salmon, F.B. Ubatuba, B.C. Weatherly, S. Moncada and J.R. Vane, "Effects of all cis-5,8,11,14,17 eicosapentaenoic acid and PGH_3 on platelet aggregation," *Prostaglandins* 18, 453-478 (1979).

(30) P. Needleman, A. Raz, M.S. Minkes, J.A. Ferrendelli and H. Sprecher, "Triene prostaglandins: Prostacyclin and thromboxane biosynthesis and unique biological properties," *Proc. Natl. Acad. Sci.* 76, 944-948 (1979).

(31) J. Dyerberg, H.O. Bang, E. Stoffersen, S. Moncada and J.R. Vane, "Eicosapentaenoic acid and prevention of thrombosis and atherosclerosis?" *Lancet* II, 117-119 (1978).

(32) H.O. Bang and J. Dyerberg, "The bleeding tendency in Greenland Eskimos," *Danish med. Bull.* 27, 202-205 (1980).

(33) C.J. Meade and J. Mertin, "Fatty acids and immunity," *Adv. Lipid Res.* 16, 127-165 (1978).

(34) U.M.T. Houtsmuller, *Proc. Golden Jubilee Internat. Congr. on EFA and Prostaglandins* (In press).

(35) F.A. Vandenheuvel, "Structure of membranes and role of lipids there in," *Adv. Lipid Res.* 9, 161-248 (1971).

(36) H.M. Sinclair, "Deficiency of essential fatty acids and atherosclerosis, etcetera," *Lancet* I, 381-383 (1956).

(37) V. Stefansson, "Cancer: Disease of Civilization?" (Hill and Wang, New York, 1960).

(38) B. Armstrong and R. Doll, "Environmental factors and cancer incidence and mortality in different countries with special reference to dietary practices," *Int. J. Cancer* 15, 617-631 (1975).

(39) Ministeriet for Gronland, "Befolkningen I Gronland 1 January 1975 samt Fodsler og Dodsfald 1 1974" (Meddelelser Fra Statistisk Kontor n. 41, 1975).

(40) Office of Population Censuses and Surveys, Ser. DH2 no. 5 (HMSO, London, 1978).

(41) V. Stefansson, "Eskimo longevity in northern Alaska," *Science* 127, 16-19 (1958).

(42) G.M. Rousselière, "Longevity among the Eskimos," *Eskimo, Churchill* 43, 13-15 (1957).

(43) A. Bertelsen, "Gronlandsk medicinsk statistik og Nosografi," *Meddelelser om Gronland* 117, 1-83 (1935).

(44) I.M. Rabinowitch, "Clinical and other observations on Canadian Eskimos in the Eastern Arctic," *Can. med. Ass. J.* 34, 487-501 (1936).

(45) E.M. Scott, I.V. Griffith, D.D. Hoskins and R.D. Whaley, "Serum cholesterol levels and blood pressure of Alaskan Eskimo men," *Lancet* II, 667 (1958).

(46) E.M. Scott, "Nutrition of Alaskan Eskimos," *Nutr. Rev.* 14, 1-3 (1956).

(47) O. Schaefer, "Medical observations and problems in the Canadian arctic," I. *Can. med. Assoc. J.* 81, 248-253 (1959); II. *Can. med. Assoc. J.* 81, 386-393 (1959).

(48) J.B. Arthaud, "Cause of death in 339 Alaskan natives as determined by autopsy," *Arch. Pathol.* 90, 433-438 (1970).

(49) S.A. Feldman, K-J. Ho, L.A. Lewis and C.B. Taylor, "Lipid and cholesterol metabolism in Alaskan Arctic Eskimos, *Arch. Pathol.* 94, 42-58 (1972).

(50) S.A. Feldman, A.H. Rubenstein, K-J. Ho, C.B. Taylor, L.A. Lewis and B. Mikkelson, "Carbohydrate and lipid metabolism in the Alaskan Arctic Eskimo," *Amer. J. clin. Nutr.* 28, 588-594 (1975).

(51) H.O. Bang, J. Dyerberg and A.B. Nielsen, "Plasma lipid and lipoprotein pattern in Greenlandic west-coast Eskimos," *Lancet* I, 1143-1145 (1971).

(52) H.C. McGill Jr., "Appraisal of cholesterol as a causative factor in atherogenesis," *Amer. J. clin. Nutr.* 32, 2632-2636 (1979).

(53) A. Elliot-Smith, "Changing patterns of disease," In *Just Consequences,* R. Waller (ed.) (Knight, London, 1971) 143-150.

(54) H.M. Sinclair, "Modern diet and degenerative diseases," In *Just Consequences,* R. Waller (ed.) (Knight, London, 1971) 85-95.

(55) T.L. Cleave, "The conception of the saccharine disease: an outline," In *Just Consequences,* R. Waller (ed.) (Knight, London, 1971), 15-33.

(56) T.L. Cleave, G.D. Campbell and N.S. Painter, *Diabetes, Coronary Thrombosis and the Saccharine Disease* (Wright, Bristol, 1969).

(57) H.M. Sinclair, "Nutritional aspects of high-extraction flour," *Proc. Nutr. Soc.* 17, 28-37 (1958).

(58) H.M. Sinclair, "Foreword," In *Multiple Sclerosis in Childhood*, E.J. Field (ed.) (Thomas, Springfield, IL, 1980) vii-xiii.

(59) R.L. Swank, "Foreword," In *Multiple Sclerosis in Childhood*, E.J. Field (ed.) (Thomas, Springfield, IL, 1980) xv and xx.

(60) V. Ramalingaswami and H.M. Sinclair, "The relation of deficiencies of vitamin A and of essential fatty acids to follicular hyperkeratosis in the rat," *Brit. J. Derm.* 65, 1-22 (1953).

(61) J.L. Rabinowitz, J.R. Gregg, J.E. Nixon and H.R. Schumacher, "Lipid composition of the tissues of human knee joints," *Clin. Orthopaedics* 143, 260-265 (1979).

(62) U. Sagild, J. Littauer, C.S. Jespersen and S. Andersen, "Epidemiological studies in Greenland 1962-1964," *Acta. med. Scand.* 179, 29-39 (1966).

(63) C.J. Mouratoff and E.M. Scott, "Diabetes mellitus in Eskimos after a decade," *JAMA* 226, 1345-1346 (1973).

(64) H.M. Sinclair, "Deficiency of essential fatty acids in lower animals," In *Essential Fatty Acids*, H.M. Sinclair (ed.) (Butterworths, London, 1958), 249-256.

(65) A.J. Houtsmuller, J. van Hal-Ferwerda, K.J. Zahn and H.E. Henkes, "Influence of different diets on the progression of diabetic retinopathy," *Prog. Fd. Nutr. Sci.* 4, 41-46 (1980).

(66) A.J. Vergroesen, E.A.M. de Deckere, F. ten Hoor and G. Hornstra, "Cardiovascular effects of linoleic acid," *Prog. Fd. Nutr. Sci.* 4, 13-25 (1980).

(67) J.M. Iacono, M.W. Marshall, R.M. Dougherty, M.A. Wheeler, J.F. Machin and J.J. Canary, "Reduction in blood pressure associated with high polyunsaturated fat diets that reduce blood cholesterol in man," *Prev. Med.* 4, 426-443 (1975).

(68) G. Triebe, H.U. Block and W. Forster, "Über das Blutdruckverhalten Kochsalz-belasteter Ratten bei Unterschiedlichem Linolsäuregehalt des Futters," *Acta Biol. Med. Germ.* 35, 1223-1224 (1976).

(69) P.J. Lewis, P. Boylan, L.A. Friedman, C.N. Hensby and I. Downing, "Prostacyclin in Pregnancy," *Brit. med. J.* 280, 1581-1582 (1980).

-7-

Testing the Lipid Hypothesis

Ronald S. Goor and Basil M. Rifkind

SUMMARY

Does lowering serum cholesterol levels reduce risk of coronary heart disease? How much does dietary cholesterol or fat intake affect serum cholesterol levels? Should cholesterol-lowering measures be advocated for the entire population, or just for individuals at high risk? These and other questions continue to challenge the cardiovascular research community, even after years of research in a variety of disciplines. In this chapter we take stock of the progress to date in research related to the lipid hypothesis (i.e., that lowering serum cholesterol reduces coronary heart disease risk), and explore the complicating factors, such as methodological shortcomings, that have thus far prevented scientists from obtaining a definitive answer on the lipid hypothesis and its related issues. The chapter concludes with a brief description of an ongoing clinical trial, the Coronary Primary Prevention Trial, which is scheduled for completion in 1983. It is hoped that the results of this trial will provide a clear answer about the validity of the lipid hypothesis.

Life expectancy in most Western industrialised countries has increased significantly, because of such factors as the introduction of antibiotics and reduced infant mortality. This increased longevity has provided the time necessary for the development of atherosclerosis. As a result of this and other factors, coronary heart disease (CHD) has become the leading cause of death in the United States, accounting for more deaths each year than cancer (#2) and accidents (#3) together. Twenty percent of the CHD deaths in the United States are in persons younger than 60 years of age. One quarter of those who suffer clinical manifestations of CHD die within 3 hours of the first symptoms. Many never reach a hospital. Another quarter die in the first few weeks after a myocardial infarction (MI). Obviously advances in intensive care in hospital are not likely to reduce mortality from sudden death. This suggests that the most fruitful approach to CHD lies with preventing rather than curing the underlying atherosclerosis.

In the last 50 years, and especially since World War II, many Western countries have become wealthier. Lifestyles have changed, with important consequences for development of CHD. Diets include more cholesterol, total fat and saturated fat and less complex carbohydrate. Jobs have become more sedentary, and, with the exception of the recent interest in jogging and other forms of exercise, leisure activity is more sedentary. Not surprisingly, obesity has become prevalent and losing weight a national preoccupation and industry.

In underdeveloped countries CHD is usually prevalent only among the affluent who eat rich foods and lead sedentary lives. CHD may be considered a disease of affluence; it is essentially absent among the poor.

The past 50 years have also witnessed great activity in the field of atherosclerosis research. Results from such different disciplines as epidemiology, biochemistry, animal experimentation, clinical observation and intervention trials have been sufficiently consistent to allow formulation of a theoretical framework for the understanding of the natural history, pathology and to a lesser extent, the treatment and management of atherosclerosis and CHD.

Of practical importance for the prevention of CHD has been the identification of risk factors–characteristics of individuals that place them at increased risk of suffering CHD. Important risk factors include heredity or family history of premature myocardial infarction, male sex, age, cigarette smoking, hypertension and elevated serum cholesterol. The latter three are modifiable. Reduction or cessation of smoking and reduction of even mild hypertension have been shown unequivocally to reduce risk. The benefits of reducing serum cholesterol levels by diet or drug remain unproven. The following policy questions related to diet and CHD prevention are currently the subjects of heated debate:

(1) Can atherosclerotic lesions be reversed, retarded or prevented by changes in the diet; and

(2) If so, should dietary intervention aimed at reducing the incidence of CHD be directed only at high risk persons or at the entire population?

Fifty years ago Anitchkow[1] was the first to address question 1 when he demonstrated that diet-induced atherosclerotic plaques in rabbit arteries could be diminished by a low fat, low cholesterol diet fed for 1½ to 2 years. Although much more evidence has been assembled since then relating dietary fat to CHD, debate still rages over the precise role of diet.

Since definitive, unequivocal evidence is not available to guide policy makers, judgement and action must be based on the incomplete, sometimes contradictory and inferential evidence now available. Opinions diverge on the proper course of action. Some have reasoned that, until the evidence unequivocally demonstrates the benefit of changing the national diet, intervention should, at most, be applied to the 5-10% of the population with severe hypercholesterolemia who are at high risk of CHD and to patients with symptoms. Others argue that, although the evidence is incomplete, the available data are sufficiently persuasive and the disease so prevalent and costly that it would be negligent to delay introducing modest and safe changes in the national diet until unequivocal data are in hand.

Before returning to a discussion of the two questions above, we review the evidence, paying particular attention to the areas in dispute.

DIETARY FAT AND BLOOD LIPIDS

Numerous studies[2] have shown that serum cholesterol levels are increased by the dietary intake of saturated fat and cholesterol, and are reduced by polyunsaturated fats. In carefully controlled metabolic ward studies of persons with normal serum cholesterol levels, Keys[3] and Hegsted[4] independently quantified the relationships between these dietary components and serum cholesterol levels. Their empirical formulae clearly show that saturated fat is twice as effective in raising serum cholesterol as polyunsaturated fat is in reducing it, i.e., it requires 2 grams of polyunsaturated fat to neutralize the elevation in serum cholesterol caused by 1 gram of saturated fat. Monounsaturated fats neither raise nor lower serum cholesterol levels and thus do not appear in the equation. Dietary cholesterol makes a positive contribution to serum cholesterol levels but is much less cholesterologenic than dietary saturated fats. The influences of cholesterol and dietary fats are independent and additive. In practice, however, cholesterol is found only in animal products that are also the main source of saturated fat.

Probably every person's serum cholesterol level is affected by dietary intake of fats and cholesterol, but individuals exhibit apparently different genetically determined responsiveness to diet. One study (Hegsted, unpublished work) has shown that a group of 13 healthy individuals on the same western-type diet (40% of calories as fat, 15% as saturated fat, 7% as polyunsaturated fat and 500 mg cholesterol per day) exhibited a normal distribution of serum cholesterol levels. The variance and mean of the curve were influenced by age and sex. Substitution of safflower oil in the diet resulted in a 21% decrease in the average serum cholesterol for the group. Individual decreases ranged from 15 to 30%. In summary, genetic variation in responsiveness to dietary constituents affecting serum lipid levels can mean that individuals with markedly different intakes of fat and cholesterol will have the same serum cholesterol level. Conversely, individuals eating identical diets can have markedly different serum cholesterol levels.

The relationship between diet and serum cholesterol is further obscured by inadequacies in methodologies for measuring dietary intakes. The commonly used 24-hour diet recall measures food consumption only during the preceding day. Numerous studies have demonstrated that not only does total energy intake for individuals vary considerably from day to day but so do the relative contributions from saturated fat, polyunsaturated fat, protein, and carbohydrate. In modern western societies the vast array of available foods allows individuals to eat totally vegetarian diets one day and diets rich in meat and dairy products the next. Daily variation in dietary intakes of individuals in a homogeneous population exceeds the variation among individuals. The 24-hour diet recall is thus an insensitive instrument for detecting differences in intake among individuals in a cross-sectional study. Finally, it is inappropriate to relate diet, as determined by 24-hour recall, to serum cholesterol levels for individuals, because the intakes and blood values reflect different time periods. Serum cholesterol levels respond slowly to dietary changes and reflect overall food consumption during the past weeks and are not noticeably affected by foods eaten during the preceding 24 hours.

Relationships between dietary intake measured by 24-hour diet recalls and serum lipids may be detected if the diets to be compared are sufficiently different and the differences are stable over time. For example, stable subgroups of vegetarians (Seventh Day Adventists) have been compared with matched co-religionists who are either non-vegetarian or who severely limit the amount of meat in their diet.[5] Serum cholesterol levels increased with increasing degrees of non-vegetarianism. Significantly lower serum cholesterols were found for vegetarians than for non-vegetarians. Dietary intakes, within a population like the United States, are not usually sufficiently different with respect to the determinants of serum cholesterol to demonstrate such relationships.

Diets differ radically among countries and these differences are relatively stable over time. In the Seven Countries Study,[6] average serum cholesterol levels were related to habitual dietary intakes in a predictable manner and with a correlation coefficient of 0.8-0.9. Fat intakes in this study ranged from 9% of calories as fat (3% saturated, 3% polyunsaturated) in Japan to 40% (18% saturated, 4.6% polyunsaturated) in the United States and 39% (22% saturated, 3% polyunsaturated) in East Finland. Comparison of the serum cholesterol distributions for Japan and East Finland reveals that an East Finn with an average or "normal" cholesterol of about 250 mg/dl would be considered severely hypercholesterolemic in Japan.

When migrants from countries with low fat, low saturated fat diets, such as Japan[7] and Italy[8] come to the United States they often develop elevated serum cholesterol. The degree of elevation is correlated with the degree of assimilation and presumably with the adoption of western diets.

The impact of dietary alteration of fat intake on serum lipids has been observed repeatedly by physicians, many of whom routinely prescribe this kind of dietary intervention. Clinical management of hypercholesterolemia usually begins with modification of the usual western diet. This involves reductions of dietary saturated fat and cholesterol and an increase of polyunsaturated fat. Adherents to the diet almost invariably experience decreased serum cholesterol levels, on average 15-25%.

The literature on dietary modification of serum cholesterol levels has been complicated by publication of results of a number of poorly conceived studies. These studies have often neglected to incorporate all of the following necessary design features: to standardize, control and monitor diets; to provide adequate time for serum cholesterol levels to equilibrate to changes in diet; to use individuals as their own controls; to vary levels to dietary constituents within ranges expected to produce changes in serum cholesterol levels. Such inadequacies may have led these studies to conclude erroneously that serum cholesterol is not affected by changes in dietary cholesterol and/or fat.

SERUM CHOLESTEROL AND CHD

There is strong and consistent evidence that implicates serum cholesterol and its main carrier low density lipoprotein (LDL) as risk factors for CHD. Such evidence comes from a variety of disciplines with different techniques and approaches, especially prospective epidemiological studies.

For example, longitudinal (prospective) studies[9] on the population of Framingham, Massachusetts have demonstrated that serum cholesterol levels are predictive of the risk of developing CHD. With levels below about 200 mg/dl, the risk of developing CHD is low. Risk rises linearly with increasing levels of cholesterol, so that subjects with cholesterol levels over 265 mg/dl have a four-fold increase in risk. The average serum cholesterol in middle-aged males in the United States is about 210 mg/dl; the 95th percentile is about 270 mg/dl.[10]

The statistical relationship between serum cholesterol and CHD almost certainly reflects an underlying causal role for serum cholesterol (and LDL) in the development of atherosclerotic plaque which gradually occludes the arterial lumen and leads to impaired blood supply to the coronary muscle, resulting in ischemic damage or a myocardial infarction.

The composition of the fats in the plaque is similar to that in the serum and is derived from the serum. Most of the serum cholesterol is carried in LDL and it is this fraction which is the source of fats in plaque. Non-human primates fed an atherogenic, hypercholesterolemic diet for 17 months develop widespread lesions.[11] The most advanced and severe of these experimentally induced lesions may be similar or even identical to those found in human atherosclerosis and in some cases may lead to myocardial infarction or sudden death.

Evidence for the role of serum cholesterol in the development of atherosclerotic plaques and CHD in humans also comes from clinical experience with patients with familial hypercholesterolemia, especially the homozygous form. Untreated homozygotes exhibit severe hypercholesterolemia, usually in excess of 600 mg/dl. They usually develop CHD and suffer fatal myocardial infarctions in the first or second decades.

International comparisons of plaque formation determined at autopsy showed that the extent and rate of development of arterial lesions are correlated with total serum cholesterol levels.[12] Autopsies performed on young soldiers (about 19 years old) killed in Korea showed that plaque formation begins early in life and is already advanced in young adults.[13]

In the Seven Countries Study[6] the Japanese ate the least cholesterologenic diet, had the lowest serum cholesterol levels and also experienced the lowest age-standardized annual incidence rates of CHD, about 15-20 per 10,000. At the other end of the spectrum, Finland, the United States and the Netherlands had CHD rates about tenfold higher: 139, 177, and 198, respectively, per 10,000. Consistent with these higher CHD rates were dietary intakes approximately fourfold higher in total fat (about 40% of calories) and 6-7 fold higher in saturated fat (17-22% of calories). Average serum cholesterol levels were also significantly higher than Japanese values. Between these two extremes were countries like Greece, Yugoslavia and Italy, with intermediate dietary intakes of fat (25-30% of calories) and saturated fat (7-14% of calories), intermediate serum cholesterol levels and intermediate CHD incidence rates: 32, 53, and 100 respectively, per 10,000.

Migrants from Japan to Hawaii and California have provided an opportunity to study the effect of adopting a western diet on serum cholesterol levels and

CHD rates.[14,15] Serum cholesterol levels are lowest in Japan, intermediate in Hawaii and highest in California. Japanese migrants living in California eat a more westernized diet (higher in saturated fat and total fat) while those living in Hawaii have dietary intakes intermediate between Japan and California. Not surprisingly, the CHD incidence rates show a gradient of increase from the low in Japan through Hawaii to the high in California.

In recent years it has become evident that prediction of CHD risk may be improved by partitioning total blood cholesterol into its various components. Total plasma cholesterol is the sum of cholesterol in the various lipoprotein fractions: very low density lipoprotein (VLDL), low density lipoprotein (LDL), and high density lipoprotein (HDL). LDL carries most (70%) of the cholesterol in the blood and is the fraction most dramatically affected by changes in dietary saturated and polyunsaturated fat and cholesterol intake. The evidence mentioned above indicates that LDL is atherogenic. The positive relation between CHD incidence rates and total serum cholesterol reflects a relation between CHD incidence and LDL levels. HDL, which seems to play a role in removing cholesterol from arterial lesions, has a strong negative correlation with incidence rates so that higher HDL levels offer protection from CHD. HDL levels are raised by alcohol consumption, estrogen use and exercise, and are low in obese subjects. Pre-menopausal women have higher average HDL levels than men of the same age. This may relate to the low CHD rates in middle-aged women and to the greater life expectancy for women than men.

WILL REDUCING SERUM CHOLESTEROL REDUCE CHD RISK?

Few scientists now question that serum cholesterol or its surrogate (LDL) level, is influenced by diet and that serum cholesterol levels constitute one of the major risk factors for CHD. What has not yet been directly proven in humans, and is still hotly debated, is whether lowering serum cholesterol values will reduce risk of developing CHD. Can the atherosclerotic lesions caused by elevated LDL levels either be prevented, retarded or reversed by reduction of serum LDL? There is much evidence to suggest that the lesions may be beneficially influenced.

As mentioned above, the first evidence of reversal of lesions came from the rabbit studies of Anitchkow 50 years ago. Since then atherosclerotic lesions have been produced by feeding atherogenic, hypercholesterolemic diets to a variety of laboratory animals from birds to non-human primates. In general, atherosclerotic lesions in experimental animals do regress following introduction of a diet low in fat or rich in polyunsaturated (linoleic acid) fats.[16] For example, monkeys fed an atherogenic diet for 17 months suffered an average luminal narrowing of almost 60%. But after 40 months on the regression diet, the luminal narrowing was only about 20% on average. However, these experimental animal lesions are imperfect models of human atherosclerosis and so it is not possible to extrapolate regression results to humans with confidence.

Definitive evidence of regression of lesions in man has been difficult to obtain because of an absence of non-invasive means of determining the degree of luminal narrowing in coronary arteries. However, suggestive though by no means conclusive evidence that a diet low in saturated fat can prevent CHD, and presumably the underlying atherosclerotic lesions, comes from studies of vegetarian Seventh Day Adventists. In a 6-year longitudinal study of 24,000 California Adventists age 35 and older, Phillips et al[17] found CHD mortality rates in Adventists ages 35-64 were 28% of the rates for the same age group of the total California population; for ages 65+, Seventh Day Adventist rates were 50% of those of their peers. As much as 50% of the reduced risk among Adventists results from their non-smoking. But the fact that non-vegetarian middle-aged Adventists had a three-fold greater risk of fatal CHD than vegetarian Adventists suggests that a large part of the reduced risk may be attributed to the vegetarian diet.

Because people do not migrate en masse from wealthy countries with atherogenic diets and high incidences of CHD to poorer countries with non-atherogenic diets and low CHD rates, there is no evidence from migrants to show that adopting a less cholesterolemic, atherogenic diet will reduce risk of CHD. But wartime food deprivations, especially of fats–in Finland, Norway, the Netherlands, the metropolitan areas of Athens and Piraeus in Greece, as well as in post-war Germany–were followed by sharp drops in CHD mortality rates within two years.[18] These lowered rates were proportional to changes in the fat content in the diet. At the same time, fat content in the U.S. diet increased and so did CHD deaths.

Epidemiological studies, such as those described above, provide clues to phenomena but cannot prove cause and effect relationships. To establish causality it is necessary to conduct a randomized, controlled clinical trial. Below we discuss the results of several dietary and drug trials aimed at testing the lipid hypothesis, which states that CHD risk can be lowered by reducing serum cholesterol either by diet or drugs.

DIET STUDIES

The ideal test of the lipid hypothesis would involve use of cholesterol-lowering diets. Positive results from such a study could be readily generalized to dietary recommendations for high risk or general populations. Certainly dietary changes offer the most benign mode of intervention.

Several studies have used dietary intervention in order to determine if long-term reduction of serum cholesterol results in lowered CHD risk. Three of these studies have provided suggestive evidence in support of the lipid hypothesis, but each was sufficiently flawed in design to preclude a definitive answer.

In the Los Angeles Veterans Administration Study,[19] 422 institutionalized men were randomized to a control diet containing 40% of calories as fat and 650 mg cholesterol. The experimental group (424 men) were fed a diet with the same fat content, but a high P/S ratio (1.7) because of substitution of vegetable oils for animal fats, and, about 365 mg cholesterol. The two groups had similar baseline blood cholesterol levels. During the eight-year study, the men in the experimental group experienced a 20% reduction in cholesterol and the control group, 7%. More dropouts in the experimental group (30% vs. 20%) may have biased the final results.

On the basis of primary endpoints (sudden death and definite myocardial infarction), there was a statistically insignificant difference in favor of the experimental group. When secondary endpoints (definite cerebral infarction, ruptured aneurysm, amputation) were included, the difference became significant. However, both groups experienced similar total mortality rates, owing in part to an increased cancer death rate in the experimental group. This increased cancer risk has raised fears that diets high in polyunsaturated fats may be carcinogenic. This observation has not been confirmed in other studies. Study power was compromised by small sample size, low adherence rates and failure to include enough young and asymptomatic patients who were the subjects with the most significant results. Nonetheless the study results provide suggestive, if not conclusive, support for the lipid hypothesis.

In the Finnish Diet Study,[20] a cholesterol-reducing diet was fed to inmates in one mental hospital from 1959-1965 and to those in another hospital from 1900-1971. The diet had a P/S ratio of 1.4 1.8 versus 0 2-0 3 of the conventional hospital diet. The diet resulted in a 12-18% reduction of blood cholesterol when compared with levels achieved in the same hospital during conventional diet feeding. Death rates during the experimental diet phase were half those in the same hospital when the conventional diet was provided.

Criticisms of this study focus on the considerable population turnover during the 12-year period. Only a small fraction of the total population at each hospital remained constant, making comparison of end point rates with control years difficult. In addition, the lack of population comparison on baseline coronary status or on potential coronary risk factors other than blood cholesterol level and age, complicated by the fact that mean cholesterol levels during the control period were substantially higher than at the start of the dietary intervention, may partially account for the difference in mortality rates. The large reduction in mortality rates in conjunction with such modest cholesterol changes raises concerns of co-interventions or other undetermined biases.

The Oslo Diet-Heart Study[21] was a secondary prevention study involving 412 men ages 30-64 years. Allocation to experimental diet (P/S ratio of 1.8) and normal control diet groups was random. The cholesterol differential achieved was 13.9%. The study patients and physicians were not blinded to treatment allocation. After 5 years of follow-up, the incidence of fatal events alone and of fatal and non-fatal events combined was significantly lower in the dietary group. There was no difference in the incidence of sudden death.

This study has been criticized for the lack of double blinding which introduces the possibility of bias resulting in potential alteration of other risk factors in the treated group; this is an especially serious flaw when non-fatal events are included. The possibility of additional interventions is strengthened by the greater reduction in event rate than is expected for such modest cholesterol lowering in a post-MI population. The Coronary Drug Project reports that blood cholesterol does not appear to be as important a risk factor in subjects who have already experienced a myocardial infarction. By 11 years of follow-up, there was no significant reduction in total CHD mortality in the treated group. Again these results offer encouraging support for the lipid hypothesis but are not conclusive.

The results of these dietary studies were sufficiently encouraging that other investigators decided to determine the feasibility of testing the lipid hypothesis by double-blind dietary intervention in a free-living population. The U.S. Diet-Heart Study[22] was designed and implemented to do this. The double-blind was maintained by use of special "look-alike" foods acquired in a commissary. The treated group achieved about a 10% reduction of cholesterol compared with the control group. Such a study would be the ideal test of the lipid hypothesis, for results would easily be generalized to dietary modification in the free-living population. However, the pilot study revealed that to provide an adequate test of the lipid hypothesis, a study would require 50,000 to 100,000 men, ages 40-59 and would cost $1 billion—and thus was not feasible.

DRUG STUDIES

Another approach to testing the lipid hypothesis involves the use of hypo-cholesterolemic drugs with or without accompanying dietary modification. Drugs offer the advantage that more substantial cholesterol lowering can be achieved than with diet alone, thus considerably improving study power. In practical terms this means fewer subjects need to be followed over a shorter period of time.

With a group of men who had suffered a myocardial infarction an average of 4 years before entry into the study, the Coronary Drug Project[23] tested the effects of four drugs (clofibrate, nicotinic acid, two dosages of D-thyroxine and two dosages of estrogen) on the incidence of reinfarction and CHD death. Although the study was well designed (e.g., double blind and randomized), it failed to provide an answer to the lipid hypothesis. A variety of reasons can be offered: cholesterol reduction achieved by the various drug regimens was probably insufficient to produce a significant decrease in event rate; participants had lower mortality than expected, probably attributable to selection of long-term survivors of a myocardial infarction who were young and relatively healthy; the extent and nature of the cardiac damage from the previous myocardial infarction was found to be a much more important risk factor for future events than the post-myocardial infarction serum cholesterol level and so reduction of serum cholesterol would not be expected to have a great influence on secondary event rates; serum cholesterol level was not a selection criterion.

Despite the failure of the Coronary Drug Project to test the lipid hypothesis adequately, it did clearly demonstrate the dangers of treating men who had had a myocardial infarction with estrogen or D-thyroxine to reduce their serum cholesterol levels. Both drops were associated with increased non-fatal and fatal event rates. These results were instrumental in the discontinuation of these therapeutic modalities. Neither clofibrate nor nicotinic acid lowered total or CHD deaths in Coronary Drug Project. Clofibrate primarily reduced serum triglyceride levels and only modestly lowered serum cholesterol levels. In addition, its use was associated with a variety of side effects, such as increased incidence of pulmonary embolism and gallstones, enlarged spleen, reduced white cell counts and hematocrits, reduced levels of bilirubin and alkaline phosphatase. Only nicotinic acid gave a hint of affecting CHD rates by reducing the rate of definite, non-fatal myocardial infarction.

The World Health Organization clofibrate study[24] was a primary prevention trial of clofibrate in free-living men in the top third of the cholesterol distribution in three European countries. An average 9% reduction in serum cholesterol levels was achieved. The treated hypercholesterolemic group experienced lower rates of non-fatal MI but similar rates of CHD death as the untreated hypercholesterolemic group. The treated group also suffered excess malignancies and deaths, especially related to the liver, biliary and intestinal systems; they also experienced an increased incidence of gallstones and cholecystectomies. Excess deaths continued to occur in the treatment group even after cessation of the drug.

In conclusion, numerous dietary and drug intervention studies have used either institutionalized or free-living populations, with or without established CHD, to determine if CHD risk can be reduced by lowering serum cholesterol levels. All these studies have failed to provide definitive evidence, owing to one or more of the following faults in study design:

(1) An insufficient number of subjects was studied to yield statistically significant numbers.

(2) The intervention was introduced too late in the life of the subjects to reduce or arrest damage developed over a lifetime.

(3) Follow-up time was insufficient.

(4) Serum cholesterol reduction was insufficient.

(5) Randomization and double-blind procedures were not used.

(6) The statistical approaches employed in data analyses were flawed.

None of these studies has provided sufficiently conclusive evidence although some resulted in suggestive evidence of benefit. Similarly, none of these studies has proved that risk of CHD is not reduced by lowering serum cholesterol.

ONGOING STUDIES

At this writing one study that may provide a conclusive answer is the Lipid Research Clinics Coronary Primary Prevention Trial (CPPT).[25] The CPPT enrolled 3,810 men with primary Type II hyperlipoproteinemia. At the outset, these men were 35-59 years old, in good health and free of any overt symptoms of CHD. All subjects were prescribed a standard diet which allowed about 400 mg cholesterol per day and a P/S ratio of approximately 0.8. In addition half of the men were prescribed 24 g/day of a bile sequestrant, cholestyramine; the other half received a placebo. Assignment of subjects to drug or placebo was done randomly within eight prognostic strata and in a double-blind manner at each of the 12 clinics. Subjects are followed for a minimum of 7 years. The primary end points are coronary death and nonfatal myocardial infarction. The CPPT is scheduled to end in July, 1983.

If the results are positive, there are good grounds to generalize from this study to predict risk reduction following dietary reduction of serum cholesterol in hypercholesterolemic men and to also extend these results to the so-called normocholesterolemic population.

The authors would like to thank Janet Bungay for editorial assistance and Beverly Neal for manuscript preparation.

REFERENCES

(1) N. Anitchkow, "Uber die Veranderungen der Kaninchenaorta bei experimenteller Cholesterinsteatose," *Beitr. Path. Anat.* 56, 537 (1913).

(2) C.J. Glueck and W.E. Connor, "Diet Coronary Heart Disease Relationships Reconnoitered," *Am. J. Clin. Nutr.* 31, 727 (1978).

(3) A. Keys, J.T. Anderson and F. Grande, "Prediction of Serum Cholesterol Responses of Man to Changes in Fats in the Diet," *Lancet* II, 959 (1957).

(4) D.M. Hegsted, R.B. McGandy, M.L. Myers and F.J. Stare, "Quantitative Effects of Dietary Fat on Serum Cholesterol in Man," *Am. J. Clin. Nutr.* 17, 281 (1965).

(5) R.O. West and O.B. Hayes, "Diet and Serum Cholesterol Levels: A Comparison Between Vegetarians and Non-vegetarians in a Seventh-Day Adventist Group," *Am. J. Clin. Nutr.* 21, 853 (1968).

(6) A. Keys (Editor), "Coronary Heart Disease in Seven Countries," *Circulation* 41, Suppl. 1, 211 pages (1970).

(7) A. Kagan, B.R. Harris, W. Winkelstein, Jr., et al, "Epidemiologic Studies of Coronary Heart Disease and Stroke in Japanese Men Living in Japan, Hawaii and California. Demographic, Physical, Dietary and Biochemical Characteristics," *J. Chronic Dis.* 27, 345 (1974).

(8) L. Katz, J. Stamler and R. Pick, *Nutrition and Atherosclerosis* (Lea and Febiger, Philadelphia, 1958).

(9) W.B. Kannel, W.P. Castelli, T. Gordon, et al, "Serum Cholesterol, Lipoproteins, and the Risk of Coronary Heart Disease: The Framingham Study," *Ann. Intern. Med.* 74, 1 (1971).

(10) The Lipid Research Clinics Population Studies Data Book, Vol. 1, *The Prevalence Study* (U.S. Dept. Health and Human Services, 1980).

(11) M.L. Armstrong and E.D. Warner, "Morphology and Distribution of Diet-induced Atherosclerosis in Rhesus Monkeys," *Arch. Path.* 92, 395 (1971).

(12) H.C. McGill, Jr. (Editor), *Geographic Pathology of Atherosclerosis* (Williams and Wilkins, Baltimore, 1968).

(13) W.F. Enos, J.C. Beyer and R.H. Holmes, "Pathogenesis of Coronary Disease in American Soldiers Killed in Korea," *JAMA* 158, 912 (1955).

(14) R.M. Worth, H. Kato, G.G. Rhoads, A. Kagan and S.L. Syme, "Epidemiologic Studies of Coronary Heart Disease and Stroke in Japanese Men Living in Japan, Hawaii and California: Mortality," *Am. J. Epidemiol.* 102, 481 (1975).

(15) M.G. Marmot, S.L. Syme, A. Kagan, H. Kato, J.B. Cohen and J. Belsky, "Epidemiologic Studies of Coronary Heart Disease and Stroke in Japanese Men Living in Japan, Hawaii and California: Prevalence of Coronary and Hypertensive Heart Disease and Associated Risk Factors," *Am. J. Epidemiol.* 102, 514 (1975).

(16) M.L. Armstrong, "Regression of Atherosclerosis," In *Atherosclerosis Reviews*, Vol. 1., Ed. R. Paoletti and A.M. Gotto (Raven Press, New York, 1976) 137.

(17) R. Phillips, F.R. Lemon, L. Beeson and J.W. Kuzma, "Coronary Heart Disease Mortality Among Seventh-Day Adventists with Differing Dietary Habits," *Am. J. Clin. Nutr.* 31, S191 (1978).

(18) H.E. Schornagel, "The Connection Between Nutrition and Mortality from Coronary Sclerosis During and After World War II," *Docum. Med. Georg. Trop.* (Amsterdam) 5, 173 (1953).

(19) S. Dayton, M.L. Pearce, S. Hashimoto et al, "A Controlled Clinical Trial of a Diet High in Unsaturated Fat in Preventing Complications of Atherosclerosis," *Circulation* 40 (Suppl. II), 1 (1969).

(20) M. Miettinen, O. Turpeinen, M.J. Karvonen et al, "Effect of Cholesterol-lowering Diet on Mortality from Coronary Heart Disease and Other Causes," *Lancet* II, 835 (1972).

(21) P. Leren, "The Effect of Plasma Cholesterol-lowering Diet in Male Survivors of Myocardial Infarction," *Acta. Med. Scand.* (Suppl.) 466, 1 (1966).

(22) "The National Diet Heart Study Final Report," National Diet Heart Study Research Group, *Circulation* 37 (Suppl. I), 1 (1968).

(23) "The Coronary Drug Project Design, Methods and Baseline Results," The Coronary Drug Project Research Group, *Circulation* 47 (Suppl. I) (1973).

(24) "A Co-operative Trial in the Primary Prevention of Ischaemic Heart Disease Using Clofibrate," Report from the Committee of Principal Investigators, *Br. Heart J.* 10, 1069 (1978).

(25) "The Coronary Primary Prevention Trial: Design and Implementation," The Lipid Research Clinics Program, *J. Chronic Dis.* 32, 609 (1979).

-8-

Role of Diet
in Lipoprotein Metabolism:
Implications for
Coronary Heart Disease

Gloria L. Vega and Scott M. Grundy

SUMMARY

The plasma lipids are transported in the form of soluble complexes known as lipoproteins. Some of the lipoproteins may play a role in atherogenesis. Following ingestion of a fatty meal, the intestine produces lipoproteins called a chylomicrons which are rich in triglyceride. Although some workers have speculated the chylomicrons are atherogenic this remains to be proven. The liver (and possibly the intestine) produces smaller lipoproteins that also are rich in triglycerides. These are very low density lipoproteins (VLDL), and again their atherogenic potential is controversial. The synthesis of VLDL is stimulated by excessive intakes of total calories, ethanol, carbohydrates and saturated fats. Another lipoprotein, low density lipoprotein (LDL), is definitely atherogenic when plasma concentrations are increased. Plasma LDL levels are enhanced by diets rich in saturated fats and cholesterol, and they are lowered by high-carbohydrate diets and polyunsaturated fats. Finally, high density lipoproteins (HDL), appear to be antiatherogenic. They are reduced by obesity and possibly by cholesterol-lowering diets, and they are increased by weight loss, exercise, and to a small extent by ethanol.

The possible relationship between diet and atherosclerosis has been a subject of great interest. If diet can affect the atherosclerotic process, we must inquire about the mechanisms for this link. Several possibilities can be considered. The most likely is that diet affects plasma lipids which in turn are atherogenic. Without doubt diet can alter plasma lipids, and it is therefore reasonable to postulate that diet can influence atherosclerosis at least indirectly. Also, we should not overlook possible connections between diet and atherosclerosis that are independent of plasma lipids. For instance, certain dietary components (e.g., oxygenated steroids and particular fatty acids) could promote atherogenesis by direct injury to the arterial wall. Also, diet might affect platelet function or other homeostatic mechanisms. Although these mechanisms deserve more investigation, the current discussion will be confined to effects of specific dietary factors on plasma lipids.

To understand the actions of different dietary constituents on plasma lipids, mechanisms for transport of lipids through the plasma must be considered. The major lipids, cholesterol, triglycerides and phospholipids are insoluble in water and thus cannot be transported as free molecules. Instead, they are solubilized through formation of lipoproteins. The latter are molecular aggregates containing specialized proteins, called apoproteins. They are amphipathic, i.e., they have a hydrophobic region that dissolves lipids and a hydrophilic region which promotes solubility in water. The lipoproteins are composed of a central core of neutral lipids (cholesterol esters and triglycerides) and a membrane-like coat of unesterified cholesterol, phospholipids, and apoproteins.

The lipoproteins are derived from either the liver or gut, and they can differ considerably in size, composition and atherogenic potential. Therefore, it may be helpful to view the relationship between diet and atherosclerosis in terms of specific lipoproteins. Thus, we will consider each lipoprotein in turn, examine evidence for its role in atherogenesis and review current information on effects of diet on its metabolism.

CHYLOMICRONS

In the intestinal lumen, dietary fats (triglycerides) are hydrolyzed into fatty acids and monoglycerides. These are taken up by the mucosa, resynthesized into triglycerides, and along with dietary cholesterol, incorporated into lipoproteins called chylomicrons. These relatively-large lipoproteins are secreted into the intestinal lymph, pass through the thoracic duct into the blood stream, and then enter capillary beds in the peripheral circulation. As chylomicrons pass through capillaries, they come into contact with an enzyme located on the surface of capillary endothelial cells. This enzyme, lipoprotein lipase, hydrolyzes the triglycerides into free fatty acids and glycerol. When lipolysis is almost complete, a residual lipoprotein, designated chylomicron remnant, returns to the circulation and is rapidly removed by the liver.

Evidence for Atherogenicity of Chylomicrons

Although chylomicrons are almost certainly less atherogenic than some of the lipoproteins to be discussed below, Zilversmit[1] has postulated that they or their products have atherogenic potential. The basis for his hypothesis can be examined briefly.

Chylomicrons are the principal carriers of dietary cholesterol, and as they are degraded some of their cholesterol may be released at the site of hydrolysis. This process might occur in two ways. First, the surfaces of large- and medium-sized arteries are covered by endothelial cells and presumably contain lipoprotein lipase; if some chylomicrons are degraded on the arteries, a portion of their cholesterol may be released and find its way into the subintimal region. This implies that cholesterol can be lost from the chylomicron and not be retained within the remnant. This latter mechanism has been shown by Fielding.[2]

Chylomicron remnants also could be atherogenic. For example, Zilversmit et al[1] demonstrated accumulation of chylomicron remnants in plasma of cholesterol-fed rabbits. The atherogenicity of dietary cholesterol for rabbits has been known for years, but Zilversmit et al[1] showed that most of the excess cholesterol in plasma of cholesterol-fed rabbits occurs as chylomicron remnants. Apparently, when the cholesterol content of chylomicrons is increased, their clearance from plasma is delayed. These remnants almost certainly contribute to arterial accumulation of cholesterol in these animals. Zilversmit[1] has speculated that a similar phenomenon may exist for man.

If atherogenesis is to some extent a postprandial phenomenon, as Zilversmit suggests,[1] then atherosclerotic coronary heart disease (CHD) may be greater in geographical areas where large quantities of fat are eaten. Indeed, several epidemiological studies have shown that the incidence of CHD is relatively low in countries where the intake of total fat is low.[3] However, as will be discussed below, these reports must be interpreted with caution.

Despite the above arguments, many investigators contend that chylomicrons probably are not atherogenic in man. They cite several types of evidence to support the opposing view; their arguments can be summarized briefly.

First, in rare diseases, such as Type I hyperlipoproteinemia, characterized by a congenital deficiency of lipoprotein lipase, enormous quantities of chylomicrons accumulate in plasma; yet patients with this disorder appear not to have accelerated atherosclerosis.[4]

Second, evidence supporting atherogenicity of chylomicron remnants in man also is relatively weak. Clearly, man does not accumulate large quantities of remnants following ingestion of dietary cholesterol as occurs in rabbits. As shown in our laboratory,[5] clearance of chylomicron remnants is very rapid in normal man, and hence their postprandial concentrations are extremely low. Therefore, it is doubtful that chylomicron remnants contribute significantly to atherosclerosis in man, as they do in cholesterol-fed rabbits.

Finally, an important question is whether CHD is more common in populations ingesting large quantities of fat than in those with low-fat diets. As indicated above, certain epidemiological studies suggest that the CHD is relatively low where intake of total fat is low.[3] Yet, its prevalence also can be low where the intake of fat is high. For example, in the seven-countries study of Keys et al,[3] intake of fat was found to be as high in Crete as in Finland and the United States (i.e., about 40% of total calories), but the prevalence of CHD in the former was much lower than in the latter two countries. Likewise, CHD in American Indians of the Southwest is low despite ingestion of a high-fat diet. The reduced CHD in Crete and in American Indians seems to be related more to a low concentration of fasting cholesterol than to the quantity of fat ingested. Therefore, data supporting atherogenicity of human chylomicrons or their remnants are weak at best.

VERY LOW DENSITY LIPOPROTEINS (VLDL)

Another category of triglyceride-rich lipoprotein is VLDL. This lipoprotein, which is smaller than the chylomicron, is made predominantly in the liver, but the intestine also can produce VLDL-sized, small chylomicrons. VLDL contains some cholesterol in addition to triglycerides, and it acquires more cholesterol esters as it circulates in plasma. The major structural apoprotein of VLDL is called apoprotein-B (apo-B), but other, more-soluble apoproteins designated "C" and "E" are also present. The triglycerides transported in VLDL are hydrolyzed by lipoprotein lipase but more slowly than those of chylomicrons; hence VLDL are cleared from plasma much slower than are chylomicrons. During lipolysis VLDL is degraded to smaller particles, VLDL "remnants". Under certain circumstances, VLDL "remnants" may be removed by the liver similar to chylomicron remnants. However, in the usual course of events, the soluble apoproteins, apo-C-I, C-II, C-III, and apo-E, are released as VLDL is catabolized, and a small particle, low density lipoprotein (LDL), containing mostly cholesterol and apo-B, is formed.

Evidence for the Atherogenicity of VLDL

VLDL is the major triglyceride-carrying lipoprotein in fasting plasma, and several epidemiological studies have claimed a positive correlation between fasting triglyceride concentration and CHD.[6] On the other hand, a direct cause-and-effect relationship between triglycerides and atherosclerosis has been difficult to show. Recently, Hulley et al[6] reviewed several ways of analyzing available data, and they show that the correlation between serum concentrations of triglycerides and CHD becomes weaker when other known risk factors, such as cholesterol, are taken into consideration. Nevertheless, their calculations do not prove that VLDL or the cholesterol carried in VLDL do not have atherogenic potential. Furthermore, there are different types of hypertriglyceridemia, with differing forms of VLDL, and it is conceivable that each type could present a different risk for CHD. Therefore, when considering the relation between VLDL and CHD, it may be worthwhile to examine the various forms of hypertriglyceridemia and what is known about the risk of each for CHD.

The most severe elevations of VLDL are found in patients with Type V hyperlipoproteinemia.[4] In this disorder, plasma triglycerides usually exceed 2000 mg/dl, and increases are found both in VLDL and chylomicrons. Although patients with Type V may be heterogenous with regard to their primary metabolic defect, most appear to have defective clearance of triglyceride-rich lipoproteins. Although CHD and peripheral vascular disease can occur in Type V patients, an increased incidence of premature atherosclerosis has not been documented with certainty. This has lead to the postulate that the large, triglyceride-rich lipoproteins found in this disorder may not be atherogenic.[7]

Pure elevations of VLDL have been designated Type IV hyperlipoproteinemia.[4] Again, this pattern may include several different metabolic defects and genetic disorders. This heterogenicity also may extend to the atherogenic potential of each disorder. Although reasons for differences in CHD risk associated with the various forms of Type IV hyperlipoproteinemia are probably complex, one factor may be differences in the size and composition of VLDL, as will be discussed below.

One form of primary Type IV hyperlipoproteinemia is *familial-hypertrigly-*

ceridemia.[4] This disorder is considered to represent an autosomal dominant trait in which patients manifest an isolated elevation of VLDL. Unfortunately, the diagnosis can be made only after extensive family screening has shown that only hypertriglyceridemia (and not hypercholesterolemia) exists in affected relatives. There is uncertainty whether patients with familial hypertriglyceridemia have premature CHD. Although early studies suggested that they have more CHD than the normal population, recent investigations have called this into question.[8] Even if their risk is somewhat increased, it seems much less than that of most other forms of hyperlipoproteinemia.

Another primary disorder, *familial combined hyperlipidemia,* likewise may be present with the Type IV pattern.[4] However, within a single family, elevations may occur in chylomicrons, VLDL and LDL, singly or in combination. Of interest, the risk for CHD can be increased even when VLDL alone are elevated.[8] Just why the Type IV pattern predisposes to CHD more in this disorder than in familial hypertriglyceridemia is not clear. One possibility is that VLDL in the former are smaller and richer in cholesterol than in the latter condition, as shown recently in our laboratory. Small, cholesterol-like VLDL may be more likely to enter the artery wall and to deposit cholesterol than larger particles mostly devoid of cholsterol.

Patients with some forms of secondary Type IV hyperlipoproteinemia also seem to be increased risk for CHD. Examples are those with diabetes mellitus and renal failure. Whether the greater risk in these diseases is related to an increased circulating VLDL remains to be determined.

Finally, another category of hypertriglyceridemia is found in patients with *Type III hyperlipoproteinemia* (dysbetalipoproteinemia). In this disorder, plasma levels of small VLDL are increased. These particles have been designated −VLDL, and they differ from normal VLDL in several ways. −VLDL are relatively low in triglycerides and "C" apoproteins, rich in cholesterol and apo-B, and have an abnormality in apo-E. Patients with dysbetalipoproteinemia are definitely at increased risk for CHD,[4] and this fact supports the concept that smaller VLDL are more atherogenic than larger ones.

The same seems to hold for experimental atherosclerosis. There is no evidence that atherosclerosis can be induced in animals when VLDL are large, rich in triglycerides, and poor in cholesterol. On the other hand, in cholesterol-fed animals, atherosclerosis develops rapidly following accumulation of small, cholesterol-containing VLDL, in plasma.

Finally, evidence that VLDL *can* contribute to atherosclerosis has been obtained from examination of atherosclerotic plaque in man.[9] Apoproteins B, C-II and C-III have been detected immunochemically suggesting the presence of VLDL or VLDL "remnants" in lesions.

Dietary Therapy of Hypertriglyceridemia

If it could be documented with certainty that some forms of hypertriglyceridemia are not associated with increased atherosclerosis, then treatment of elevated triglycerides obviously would not be needed. On the other hand, even if risk for CHD is not increased strikingly, a reduction in triglycerides by dietary means may be prudent. The use of drug therapy is another matter and depends on a judgement of the relative benefits and risks.

In Type V hyperlipoproteinemia, dietary therapy usually is warranted for reasons other than to prevent atherosclerosis. When triglycerides are greatly elevated by hyperchylomicronemia, acute pancreatitis may occur. To prevent pancreatitis, circulating chylomicrons can be lowered by decreasing daily fat intake to 30 gm or less. Since many patients with Type V patterns are obese, a reduction of fat intake can be combined with caloric restriction; this will reduce both chylomicrons and VLDL. If dietary measures fail to control hyperchylomicronemia, consideration can be given to drug therapy (e.g., nicotinic acid or clofibrate) to prevent pancreatitis. The use of these drugs to retard atherosclerosis is more controversial because the initial risk for CHD is not known. Nonetheless, drug therapy may be justified if the patient has evidence of premature atherosclerosis or if it exists in the family.

Familial hypertriglyceridemia presents a similar dilemma for therapy. If the decision is made to treat this disorder, caloric restriction should be tried, particularly if significant obesity is present; a decreased intake of calories will curtail the synthesis of VLDL. Some patients with hypertriglyceridemia of this type are extremely sensitive to alcohol, and respond to abstinence with a significant reduction of triglycerides.

Since patients with familial combined hyperlipidemia are at high risk for CHD, an attempt to lower triglycerides seems justified. If the patient is obese, he should be urged to loose weight. Replacement of fat with carbohydrate should be avoided because of the phenomenon of carbohydrate-induced hypertriglyceridemia.[10] Where possible, polyunsaturated fat should be used in place of saturated fat because the former has a VLDL-lowering action.[11] If lipids cannot be normalized in these patients, drug therapy must be considered.

Diet alteration can sometimes be highly effective in Type III hyperlipoproteinemia. Caloric restriction is most effective if the patient is obese. Also, saturated fats and dietary cholesterol should be decreased, and polyunsaturated fats can be increased. Nonetheless, most patients with this disease require drug therapy (e.g., clofibrate) to normalize their plasma lipids.

LOW DENSITY LIPOPROTEINS

Most of the cholesterol in human plasma is transported as cholesterol esters in LDL. As indicated above, LDL is thought to be derived mainly from VLDL. LDL appears to be a major source of cholesterol for tissue other than the liver. Many cells of the body have high-affinity receptors for LDL; these receptors bind this lipoprotein LDL leading to its internalization and catabolism in lysosomes. Cholesterol esters are hydrolyzed, and the resulting unesterified cholesterol is released into the cytoplasm; here it can serve as a component of cell membranes, suppress the cells own synthesis of cholesterol, or be reesterified and stored within vacuoles as cholesterol esters.

Evidence for the Atherogenicity of LDL

The best evidence for the atherogenic potential of LDL is found in the high risk of patients with hypercholesterolemia. There are several forms of hypercholesterolemia associated with elevated LDL levels, and in general, risk for CHD rises with increasing cholesterol concentrations. The major categories of hypercholesterolemia and their relative risks for CHD can be reviewed briefly.

Familial hypercholesterolemia is characterized by a marked increase in plasma cholesterol to the range of 300 to 500 mg/dl. LDL-cholesterol is usually over 200 mg/dl. The disease is associated with very severe atherosclerosis, and CHD commonly becomes manifest in the 20's or 30's. Tendon xanthomas are frequent. The disorder is inherited as an autosomal dominant, and the primary defect resides in a reduced uptake of LDL by tissues caused by a decrease in the number of LDL-receptors. Familial hypercholesterolemia is one of the most common inborn errors of metabolism with an incidence of about 1 per 500 in the population.

As indicated above, patients with *familial combined hyperlipidemia* may have an increase in LDL as well as VLDL. Patients with this form of hypercholesterolemia are prone to premature atherosclerosis, but less so than with familial hypercholesterolemia. In the former hyperlipidemia does not appear as early in life or with the degree of severity found in the latter. Cholesterol concentrations are usually in the range of 275 to 350 mg/dl.

Another group of patients have increased LDL without evidence of a monogenic inheritance. They are said to have polygenic hypercholesterolemia. Several members of a family may have hypercholesterolemia, or it can occur sporadically in one family member without its being present in any of the others. Concentrations of total cholesterol and LDL in polygenic hypercholesterolemia are about the same as in familial combined hyperlipidemia. Presumably, the risk for CHD is also about the same.

Probably the most common form of hypercholesterolemia is dietary-induced hypercholesterolemia. Cholesterol concentrations generally are increased only mildly (e.g., total cholesterol = 200-250 mg/dl). This condition almost certainly contributes greatly to the high incidence of CHD in our society. Considerable epidemiological evidence shows that people with cholesterol levels in the range of 200 to 250 mg/dl are at significantly greater risk for CHD than those with concentrations below 200 mg/dl. Although genetic factors may play a role in raising cholesterol to this range in some people, dietary factors are probably the major cause. In other words, by moderate dietary alteration, it should be possible to reduce cholesterol levels to below 200 mg/dl.

Several animal models have been used to examine the relation between LDL concentrations and atherosclerosis. Increased LDL levels can be increased by cholesterol feeding, and high-cholesterol diets are atherogenic in rabbits, monkeys, swines, pigeons, rats, and dogs. Although hypercholesterolemia can be induced in these animals, the elevated, cholesterol-rich lipoproteins do not always resemble human LDL. In some species the main increase in cholesterol occurs in VLDL; in others, LDL particles are abnormally large.[12] Frequently, an excess accumulation of apo-E occurs in LDL and VLDL. Thus, while animal studies show that elevated plasma cholesterol can cause atherosclerosis, they provide only indirect evidence that human LDL are atherogenic.

More direct evidence for the atherogenicity of LDL in man has been obtained by examination of human atherosclerotic lesions. Immunochemical probes have demonstrated the presence of LDL components in these lesions.

For instance, two forms of apo-B (i.e., tightly bound and loosely bound forms) have been identified in plaques;[12] these were thought to be derived from LDL.

DIETARY THERAPY OF HYPERCHOLESTEROLEMIA (ELEVATED LDL)

Genetic Hypercholesterolemia

In the genetic forms of hypercholesterolemia (e.g., familial hypercholesterolemia, familial combined hyperlipidemia, and polygenic hypercholesterolemia), dietary therapy alone is rarely sufficient to normalize LDL levels. Although diets low in saturated fats and cholesterol and high in polyunsaturated fats can be employed, they are usually inadequate to reduce total cholesterol below 200 to 250 mg/dl, and drug therapy almost always is required. The pharmacological therapy of these disorders is beyond the scope of this chapter, but we should emphasize that they should not be treated inadequately by dietary means alone.

Diet-Induced Hypercholesterolemia

The greatest potential for dietary therapy of hypercholesterolemia would seem to be for people with mild elevations of total plasma cholesterol (200 to 250 mg/dl). Indeed, for most people, these mildly-elevated levels are probably due to excessive intake of certain dietary constituents (saturated fats, cholesterol, and total calories). On the basis of equations developed by Keys et al[13] and Hegsted et al,[14] effects of different nutrients on plasma cholesterol can be calculated. For example, the current U.S. diet contains about 40% of total calories as fat, and cholesterol intake is about 500 mg/day. Fat calories include approximately 18% as saturated fats, 16% as monounsaturated fats, and 6% as polyunsaturated fats. The American Heart Association and the Senate Select Committee on Nutrition have recommended that the U.S. population reduce cholesterol to 300 mg/day and fat intake to 30%; these groups recommend an equal distribution of saturated, monounsaturated and polyunsaturated fats, i.e., 10%:10%:10%. The reduction in fat calories from 40 to 30% would require a replacement of 10% of calories by carbohydrates. Also, it is suggested that weight be reduced to the ideal range. Using the equations of Keys et al[13] and Hegsted et al[14] it can be shown that this dietary change would reduce plasma cholesterol to near or below 200 mg/dl in patients with diet-induced hypercholesterolemia. Unfortunately, it has not been proven that such an induced reduction in plasma cholesterol will decrease CHD; nevertheless, since people with diet-induced hypercholesterolemia have about twice the risk for CHD as those with cholesterol levels below 200 mg/dl, a dietary modification would seem prudent.

Diet Change in People Without Hypercholesterolemia

An important question is whether diet change should be recommended for those whose cholesterol levels are below 200 mg/dl. For example, would a reduction of plasma cholesterol from 190 to 150 mg/dl by dietary change reduce the risk for CHD? To date, on the basis of existing epidemiological data, there is no evidence to support such a change. From the combined data of several epidemiological studies in the U.S.,[15] a graded relation between plasma cholesterol levels and CHD could not be demonstrated when cholesterol was below 200 mg/dl. Therefore, there seems little justification, on scientific grounds alone, to recommend alteration in diet for these people.

HIGH DENSITY LIPOPROTEINS (HDL)

HDL, like LDL, participates in cholesterol transport. At least 4 classes of HDL have been isolated from plasma: HDL_3, HDL_2, HDL_1, and HDL-I. The origins of the components of plasma HDL are complex. Some are secreted directly by the liver and intestine; other are derived from the catabolism of chylomicrons and VLDL as well as from other enzymatic reactions in plasma. The primary apoproteins of circulating HDL are apo A-I and apo A-II. These are synthesized by the intestine and probably by the liver. Another apoprotein associated with HDL is apo E which comes mainly from the liver. The phospholipids of HDL are obtained either by direct secretion from liver or intestine, or as a product of the catabolism of triglyceride-rich lipoproteins. Unesterified cholesterol of HDL is partially derived from extrahepatic tissues. Also, it can come from the surface coat of triglyceride-rich lipoproteins during their metabolism. In the plasma there is an enzyme that esterifies most of the unesterified cholesterol of HDL. This enzyme is called lecithin-cholesterol acyl transferase (LCAT). HDL_3, the smallest of the HDL particles, is the primary substrate of LCAT, and apo A-I is the cofactor for this enzyme. As the reaction progresses, HDL_3 is probably converted to the larger HDL_2. The major function of HDL is apparently to carry cholesterol from one site to another. For example, it may play a role in transport of cholesterol from peripheral tissues to liver. Metabolism of HDL seems to be related to that of other lipoproteins. Cholesterol esters of HDL may be transferred to LDL and VLDL, and in turn, some components of HDL may be derived from catabolism of these lipoproteins. The fates of all components of HDL are not known. Whether this lipoprotein is removed predominately by the liver or by peripheral tissues remains to be determined.

Evidence for the Antiatherogenicity of HDL

Several epidemiological studies have demonstrated an inverse correlation between HDL-cholesterol and CHD.[16,17] This finding has prompted a more systematic study of HDL since this lipoprotein might in some way protect against development of atherosclerosis. Whether high HDL is directly antiatherogenic or merely reflects the actions of other factors on cholesterol metabolism is not clear. One possibility is that high HDL signifies a more efficient metabolism of other lipoproteins–LDL, VLDL, or chylomicrons. Something of the role of HDL in overall lipid metabolism may be learned from the study of diseases in which HDL is deficient. Thus, a brief digression to consider these conditions seems in order.

One example is Tangiers disease in which HDL is virtually absent. In this disease cholesterol accumulates in many tissues and particularly in the reticulo-endothelial system. The metabolic defect responsible for the low HDL in this disorder has not been determined. However, as a consequence of reduced HDL, the metabolism of other lipoproteins is deranged. VLDL exhibits an abnormal electrophoretic mobility while LDL has a high content of triglycerides and reduced cholesterol ester. Also, the removal of chylomicron remnants appears to be defective. Whether lesser reductions of HDL produce more subtle abnormalities in lipoprotein metabolism that could facilitate accumulation of cholesterol in tissues needs to be determined.

Another disorder affecting HDL metabolism is hereditary LCAT deficiency. In this disorder large quantities of unesterified cholesterol are present in plasma because of a failure in esterification. Since cholesterol esterification does not occur in HDL, the normal exit of cholesterol from plasma may be impaired. This again suggests that HDL is involved in an important way in the metabolism of other lipoproteins.

Thus, the role of high HDL in protection against CHD is not clear. It might directly promote the efflux of cholesterol from tissues, or it could affect the net mass of cholesterol delivered to tissues by affecting the metabolism of other lipoproteins.

Effects of Diet on HDL

The effects of at least 5 different alterations in diet on metabolism of HDL have been examined. These include diets rich in carbohydrate, polyunsaturated fats, cholesterol, ethanol, as well as caloric restriction. Two groups of investigators have reported that high-carbohydrate diets decrease HDL-cholesterol.[18,19] In one of these studies, Blum et al[20] indicated that HDL reduction is associated with a fall in ratios of HDL_2/HDL_3 and of apo A-I/A-II compared to a normal diet. Almost identical changes have been reported by Shepherd et al,[20] for diets very rich in polyunsaturated fats. These modifications have been found only for radical changes in diet composition, and lesser changes may not similarly affect concentrations of HDL.[21,22] Whether decreases in HDL-cholesterol, which may occur with various cholesterol-lowering diets, enhance the risk for CHD is unknown.

Obese patients often have a low HDL-cholesterol, and weight reduction can return their levels to normal. A low HDL-cholesterol in obesity may be explained by 2 mechanisms. First, if VLDL-triglycerides are elevated, HDL contains more triglycerides at the expense of cholesterol. Upon weight loss, HDL-triglyceride decreases while the cholesterol content is restored to normal. Second, other undefined factors associated with obesity also reduce total concentrations of HDL; again caloric restriction seems to raise HDL towards normal. In our opinion, this rise in HDL-cholesterol could be the most important action of caloric restriction on prevention of CHD. Of interest, the rise in HDL-cholesterol produced by caloric restriction can be augmented with vigorous exercise.

Other dietary factors may increase HDL-cholesterol as well. For example, ethanol consumption apparently enhances HDL levels. The mechanism of this action is not known, and whether the increase will be protective against CHD remains to be determined. Another way whereby cholesterol in HDL can be increased is by cholesterol feeding. In animal models cholesterol feeding results in the appearance of a unique lipoprotein, HDL_c. This particle is enriched in cholesterol ester; it has apo E and apo A-I as its major protein components, and its hydrated density resides between HDL_2 and LDL. The appearance of a similar lipoprotein has been described in humans during cholesterol feeding.[23] It cannot be assumed however that an increase in HDL-cholesterol during cholesterol feeding will be protective against CHD; in fact, the abnormal HDL_c could be atherogenic because of its high content of apo E which behaves similarly to apo B in tissue culture.

REFERENCES

(1) D.B. Zilversmit, *Circulation* 60, 473 (1979).
(2) C.J. Fielding, *J. Clin. Invest.* 62, 141 (1978).
(3) A. Keys (ed), *Circulation* 42, Suppl. 1 (1970).
(4) D. Fredrickson, J.L. Goldstein and M.S. Brown, in: *Metabolic Basis of Inherited Diseases,* J.B. Stanbury, J.B. Wyngaarden, D.S. Fredrickson (eds) 605 (1978).
(5) S.M. Grundy and H.Y.I. Mok, *Metabolism* 25, 1225 (1976).
(6) S.B. Hulley, R.H. Roseman, R.D. Bawol and R.J. Brand, *New Engl. J. Med.* 302, 1383 (1980).
(7) J.D. Brunzell, H.G. Schrott, A.G. Motulsky and E.L. Bierman, *Metabolism* 25, 313 (1976).
(8) H.F. Hoff, C.L. Heideman, R.L. Jackson, R.J. Bayardo, H.S. Kim and A.M. Gotto, Jr., *Circ. Res.* 37, 72 (1979).
(9) J.L. Knittle and E.H. Ahrens, *J. Clin. Invest.* 43, 485 (1964).
(10) S.M. Grundy, *J. Clin. Invest.* 55, 169 (1975).
(11) L.L. Rudel, L.L. Pihs and C.A. Nelson, *J. Lipid Res.* 18, 211 (1977).
(12) H.F. Hoff, C.L. Heideman, J.W. Gaubatz, J.L. Titus and A.M. Gotto, Jr., *Atherosclerosis* 30, 263 (1978).
(13) A. Keys, J.T. Anderson and F. Grande, *Metabolism* 14, 776 (1965).
(14) D.M. Hegstead, R.B. McGandy, M.L. Nyu and F.J. Stare, *Am. J. Clin. Nutr.* 17, 281 (1965).
(15) D.P. Barr, E.M. Russ and H.S. Eder, *Am. J. Med.* 11, 480 (1951).
(16) N.E. Miller, D.S. Thelle and O.H. Forde, *Eur. J. Clin. Invest* 8, 1979 (1978).
(17) D.E. Wilson and R.S. Lees, *J. Clin. Invest.* 51, 1051 (1972).
(18) C.B. Blum, R.I. Levy, S. Eisenberg, M. Hall, III, R.H. Goebel and M. Berman, *J. Clin. Invest.* 60, 795 (1977).
(19) A. Nicholl, N.E. Miller and B. Lewis, *Adv. Lipid Res.* 17, 92 (1980).
(20) J. Shepherd, C.J. Packard, J.R. Patsch, A.M. Gotto, Jr. and D.P. Tauton, *J. Clin. Invest.* 61, 1582 (1978).
(21) R.W. Mahley, T.P. Bersot, T.L. Innerarity, A. Lipson and S. Margolis, *Lancet* 2 (8094), 807 (1978).
(22) R.W. Mahley, T.L. Innerarity, *J. Biol. Chem.* 252, 3980 (1977).
(23) R.W. Mahley, T.L. Innerarity, R.E. Pitas, K.H. Weisgraber, J.H. Brown and E. Gross, 252, 7279 (1977).

-9-

Diabetes Mellitus and Nutrition

Richard J. Jarrett

SUMMARY

Of the two major varieties of diabetes (Type I or insulin-dependent diabetes; Type II or non-insulin-dependent diabetes) only in Type II is there evidence of a nutritional component in its aetiology. Although claims have been made for an excess of sucrose and a deficiency of chromium as aetiological factors, the evidence is slender. The major association of diabetes prevalence both within and between populations is the frequency and degree of adiposity. However, as Type II diabetes occurs in relatively lean individuals, albeit at low frequency, there must be other genetic and/or environmental, factors involved. Tropical or malnutrition diabetes may be related to undernutrition in infancy and childhood. The variant associated with pancreatic calcification is most often found in cassava eating populations and may be caused by a combination of protein deficiency and cyanide intoxication. Coronary heart disease, a major cause of morbidity and mortality in many diabetic populations, is relatively uncommon in some, e.g., Japan. This relative freedom may be due to the usual diet in these populations, which is characterised by a proportionately high complex carbohydrate and a low fat intake.

Many lines of evidence have led to the inescapable conclusion that diabetes mellitus is a genetically and clinically heterogeneous group of disorders that share hyperglycaemia or glucose intolerance as the phenotypic expression. The evidence is summarised in Table I. Furthermore, epidemiological studies have emphasised the unsatisfactory nature of criteria for diagnosing diabetes, in particular the confusion surrounding the use of glucose tolerance tests. The lack of internationally agreed diagnostic criteria and a system of classification prompted the National Diabetes Data Group of the National Institute of Health to set up an international working group. This body reported its proposals[1] in 1979 and they have since been broadly adopted by the Expert Committee of the World Health Organisation. Diabetes is classified under three headings: Type I, or insulin-dependent diabetes mellitus (Table II); Type II, or non-insulin-dependent diabetes mellitus (Table III); and other types of diabetes (Table IV).

Table I: Evidence Favouring the View that Diabetes Mellitus Is a Heterogeneous Condition

(1) The existence of more than 30 distinct, usually rare, disorders in which glucose intolerance is an associated phenomenon.

(2) Ethnic variations in diabetes prevalence and clinical type of diabetes.

(3) Genetic and immunological studies which show differences between classical "juvenile-onset" diabetes and "adult-onset" diabetes.

(4) Demonstration of a variety of diabetes with onset at young age, but not insulin dependent, in which the inheritance appears to be autosomal dominant.

(5) Genetic heterogeneity in animal models of diabetes.

Table II: Type I, Insulin-Dependent Diabetes Mellitus

The first subclass of diabetes, Type I or insulin-dependent diabetes mellitus (IDDM), is usually characterised clinically by abrupt onset of symptoms, insulinopenia and dependence on injected insulin to sustain life, and proneness to ketosis. Classically, this type of disease occurs in juveniles, and it was formerly termed juvenile diabetes. However, it can be recognised and become symptomatic for the first time at any age; hence, diagnosis based on age at onset is inappropriate. In addition to the ketosis-prone stage, this type of diabetes can also be recognised in a preketosis-prone stage. For example, prospective testing in siblings of insulin-dependent diabetics has disclosed patients with normal fasting plasma glucose (FPG) levels but with abnormal glucose tolerance who progress rapidly to the ketotic form, usually within two years after recognition, but occasionally after longer periods of time. IDDM appears to be heterogeneous in terms of genetics and environmental factors that precipitate the disease. Genetic determinants are thought to be important in most patients, as expressed by the associated increased or decreased frequency of certain histocompatibility antigens (HLA) on chromosome 6. Abnormal immune responses and autoimmunity are also thought to play an aetiologic role, and islet cell antibodies are frequently present at diagnosis in this type of diabetes.

Table III: Type II, Non-Insulin-Dependent Diabetes Mellitus

The second subclass of diabetes, Type II or non-insulin-dependent diabetes mellitus (NIDDM), frequently presents with minimal or no symptoms referable to the metabolic aberrations of diabetes. Patients with NIDDM are not dependent on insulin for prevention of ketonuria and are not prone to ketosis. However, they may require insulin for correction of symptomatic, or persistent, fasting hyperglycaemia if this cannot be achieved with the use of diet or oral agents. Such patients may develop ketosis under special circumstances, such as severe stress precipitated by infections or trauma. There may be normal levels of insulin, mild insulinopenia, or above normal level of insulin associated with insulin resistance. The whole range of insulin responses to glucose from low to supranormal has been found in patients of this subclass, many of whom do not have fasting hyperglycaemia. Patients with NIDDM may be asymptomatic for years or decades and show only slow progression of the disease. However, the typical chronic associations and complications of diabetes, namely macroangiopathy, microangiopathy, neuropathy, and cataracts, may be seen in this type. NIDDM undoubtedly is also heterogeneous in nature. Although in most patients who develop NIDDM the onset is after age 40, the NIDDM type also occurs in young persons who do not require insulin and are not ketotic. Consequently, age at onset is again not recommended as a criterion by which to classify an individual, and the terms adult-onset diabetes and variations of this phrase, should be abandoned as classifying terms.

NIDDM also has a genetic basis, which appears to be stronger than in IDDM, as evidenced by a more frequent familial pattern of occurrence. Indeed, included within this type are families in whom diabetes presents in children, adolescents, and adults in which autosomal dominant inheritance has been well established (formerly referred to as maturity-onset-type diabetes of the young, or MODY). Environmental factors superimposed on genetic susceptibility are undoubtedly involved in onset of the NIDDM types. Intake of excessive calories leading to weight gain and obesity is probably an important factor in its pathogenesis. In persons with this type of diabetes, characteristic aggregation of HLA types and islet cell antibodies have not been found.

Table IV: Other Types of Diabetes

In this subclass, diabetes forms part of certain other conditions and syndromes that often have many clinical features not generally associated with the diabetic state. In some instances the co-occurrence of glucose intolerance and the other features is known to be aetiologically related. In others, the frequency of co-occurrence indicates that there is an, as yet unknown, causal relationship. Thus, this subclass has been divided according to the known or suspected aetiological relationships. For example, diabetes may be secondary to (1) pancreatic disease or removal of pancreatic tissue, (2) endocrine diseases such as acromegaly, Cushing's syndrome, phaeochromocytoma, glucagonoma, somatostatinoma, and primary aldosteronism, or (3) the administration of certain hormones, drugs, and chemicals that cause hyperglycaemia. Diabetes may also be associated with defects of insulin receptors, which may be caused by either abnormalities in numbers or affinity of insulin receptors or antibodies to receptors with or without associated immune disorders. Diabetes (or carbohydrate intolerance) is found in increased frequency with a large number of genetic syndromes. Finally, this class contains room for certain special types of diabetes that occur only under specific, well-described environmental and clinical conditions, e.g., diabetes associated with malnourished populations.

Although environmental as well as genetic factors are important in determining the onset of Type I diabetes, there is little to suggest that nutrition plays any significant role. The evidence that does exist is circumstantial. Thus, rates of Type I diabetes with onset in the first two decades of life have been comparatively low in certain countries, e.g., Japan and Israel[2,3] and in the black inhabitants of the U.S.A.[4] Incidence rates have increased in recent years during which many changes, including nutritional ones, have taken place in these populations. It is conceivable, but by no means proven, that an increased calorie intake in infancy and childhood might add to the risk of developing diabetes in children with a genetic predisposition.

An association between obesity and Type II diabetes has been apparent for many years. In a classic paper[5] Joslin showed not only that diabetes was very much more common in the obese but also that it was more common in those of average weight than in people who had always been especially lean. Many studies within population groups, including prospective investigations, have confirmed the association (see Reference 4). In addition there are many studies which demonstrate a lowering of blood glucose levels or an improvement in glucose tolerance following weight loss. West and his colleagues[6-8] have carried out standardised international studies of diabetes prevalence in the context of nutrition and adiposity. In ten populations studied, diabetes frequency in adults (35 + years of age) was highly correlated with "average fatness", measured as the percentage of standard weight. Within population groups, for example in Central America, diabetes was three times as common in people who were slightly to moderately obese compared to people near standard weight. Amongst the several ethnic groups in these studies differences in diabetes prevalence were very small after adjustment for differences in adiposity.

The effect of obesity has been shown most dramatically by the appearance of diabetes in almost epidemic proportions in several populations. The two most extreme examples are the Pima Indians of Arizona[9] and the inhabitants of the island of Nauru in the Central Pacific.[10]

The Pima Indians and their ancestors have lived in the Arizona desert for two thousand years, cultivating crops with the help of water from the Gila River. For many years their health care has been in the hands of the Indian Medical Service and it would appear that diabetes was an uncommon condition before the Second World War. In 1963 it was noted that many of the adult Pima had diabetes and in 1965 a systematic study of diabetes was begun. It was subsequently found that diabetes was extraordinarily frequent—with about half of those aged 45 years and above having the disease.

Nauru has several claims to fame. It is the smallest republic in the world and its inhabitants have the highest per capita income in the world–thanks to the fact that most of the surface of Nauru contains high-grade phosphate ore. The Nauruans have also been systematically studied and a prevalence of diabetes almost as high as that among the Pima Indians has been discovered.

Both the Pima Indians and the Nauruans have radically changed their mode of life in the past few decades. One of the consequences of these changes is that both groups have become very obese. In the Pima the average energy intake is over 3000 kcal and in Nauru it is over 6000! The major items in the Pima diet are pinto beans, tortillas made from wheat flour and chilli peppers.

They eat less sucrose than the general population of the United States, but about the same proportion of saturated and unsaturated fats.

The Pima and the Nauruans are not the only people who have experienced an explosive increase in the frequency of diabetes. Several other North American Indian tribes, groups of Polynesians, Asian Indians in South Africa and Australian Aborigines have all been similarly affected. This mid- to late-twentieth-century phenomenon affecting people emerging from subsistence economies has led the American geneticist, Neel, to propose his 'thrifty gene' hypothesis.[11] Neel suggested that subjects from populations which had been subjected to fluctuations of food supplies and who might have experienced periods of abundance alternating with periods of famine, might have developed a propensity to store food as adipose tissue in times of abundance and, at the same time, maintain normal blood sugar levels. This trait might offer selective advantages for survival during a period of famine, in which case it would become common throughout the population by genetic selection. Given perpetual 'abundance', however, the trait is disadvantageous, leading to obesity and thence to diabetes. While the theory is obviously untestable, it is a plausible explanation of the observed phenomena. There are parallels in the animal world. Certain desert animals–the Egyptian sand-rat, the Chinese hamster, the tuco-tuco–when transferred to a laboratory or a zoo and fed a standard diet tend to develop diabetes.

The place of diet in causing Type II diabetes has been debated for many years. In the 1930s, Himsworth[12] collected data on food consumption and diabetes mortality rates from many countries and came to the conclusion that the highest diabetes rates occurred in those countries with relatively high fat and low carbohydrate diets. He adduced experimental support for this by demonstrating that a reduced carbohydrate intake led to impaired glucose tolerance –measured by the blood glucose response to an oral or intravenous glucose load. The fat hypothesis has been challenged by a number of workers, in particular Yudkin, who has shown that fat and sucrose consumption within countries is highly correlated. Yudkin has also claimed that, when national diabetes mortality rates in the mid-1950s are related to average national sugar and fat intakes about twenty years earlier, there is a better correlation with sugar intake than with fat intake.[13] Cleave has put forward a hypothesis suggesting that a large number of diseases are predominantly caused by the change to high consumption of refined carbohydrate, predominantly sucrose, and that diabetes is one of these conditions.[14] The evidence is largely epidemiological in nature, based upon rates of diabetes in population groups which have changed their dietary habits. The most widely quoted example is that of the Yemenite Jews who had emigrated to Israel. It was observed that the frequency of diabetes in newly arrived immigrants was very low–of the order of 0.06%. In similar immigrants, settled in the country for twenty-five years or more, the frequency was 2.6%, a fortyfold difference, presumably due to environmental factors. It was claimed by Cohen and his colleagues, who carried out the study, that the major change in dietary habits was an increase in sucrose consumption and that this was the cause of the increased frequency of diabetes.[15]

The problem of evaluating studies of this kind is that many changes accompany 'acculturation', amongst them being, usually, an increase in the frequency of obesity, which in most studies is the most impressive correlate of diabetes frequency. Another Israeli study provides more direct evidence against sucrose being a specifically diabetogenic factor. In a large prospective study of Israeli Civil Servants, dietary information was collected on individuals prior to the development of diabetes. Those who ultimately developed diabetes during the period of observation actually consumed *less* sugar on average than those who remained non-diabetics. The confounding factors are again obesity and energy expenditure, for on average fat people eat less of all energy-containing foods than thin people.[16]

West[17] has reviewed the extensive literature concerning the possible relationship between specific constituents (e.g., carbohydrate, fat, sucrose) and the aetiology of diabetes. His conclusion, which I share, is that while it remains possible that some individuals may be specifically sensitive to an excess of a particular dietary constituent, it is adiposity–plus duration of adiposity–however caused, which is the major environmental factor involved in the genesis of Type II diabetes. Other nutrients have been implicated. Deficiency of chromium leads to glucose intolerance in rats and this observation led to studies in man, reviewed by Hambidge.[18] Epidemiological investigations of the relationship between diabetes, tissue chromium levels and chromium availability in food have not revealed any consistent relationships. Claims have been made that chromium supplements have led to improvement in glucose tolerance in malnourished infants and in elderly subjects. However, these studies are open to criticism concerning their methodology. More information is required before the hypothesis that chromium deficiency is responsible for some human diabetes can be properly evaluated.

The subject of dietary fibre is currently of considerable interest and research, though it cannot be considered as entirely new. As long ago as 1918 Dr. John Kellogg, 'father' of the breakfast cereal, warned of the dangers of "concentrated" foods and advocated diets containing generous amounts of fruits, cereals and bran.[19] Trowell[20] has reviewed the evidence concerning the hypothesis that a deficiency of dietary fibre might contribute to the genesis of Type II diabetes. Evidence in favour is chiefly epidemiological and circumstantial in nature.

A major problem in evaluating dietary fibre as a possible protective factor is that within populations fibre consumption is associated, both positively and negatively, with a number of other factors also implicated in the aetiology of diabetes, e.g., adiposity, exercise, total carbohydrate intake, fat consumption and sucrose consumption. As adiposity has such a strong relationship with diabetes, the contribution of other factors, even if it exists, would be difficult to determine. A number of studies have been performed of diets modified by the addition of various fibre sources and many of these have been reviewed by Andersen and Chen.[21] There is little doubt that the supplementation of low fibre diets by various plant fibres can improve glucose tolerance or, in diabetics, reduce post-prandial blood glucose levels. There are differences, however, in the responses obtained with different foods or with different fibres. Thus in one study of non-diabetics, meals calculated to provide 50 g glucose were administered.[22] Plasma glucose and insulin responses to dextrose and potatoes were similar.[23] Levels of glucose and insulin were lower after meals containing rice, corn or bread as the carbohydrate source.

In another study of the effects of fibre on glucose tolerance in normal men, a low fibre basal diet (1 g crude fibre/100 kcal) was compared with a similar diet including bread supplemented for one month with 26 g of red spring wheat, soft white wheat bran, corn bran, soybean hulls, freeze-dried apple powder, or freeze-dried carrot powder. Only the two wheat brans failed to produce significant improvement in glucose tolerance, though the two powders actually contained less fibre.

There is increasing experience of the use of high carbohydrate/high fibre diets in diabetics. Such diets, if isocaloric, also tend to reductions in plasma cholesterol levels,[24] so that there may be potential benefit both in terms of glucose and lipid metabolism. Whether or not the relatively low fibre diets of modern societies actually predispose to diabetes, in the absence of adiposity, must remain an open question at present.

MALNUTRITION DIABETES

In countries lying between the Tropics of Cancer and Capricorn a form of diabetes has been recognised which differs from the two major types already considered. Affected individuals develop diabetes in adolescence or as young adults, are characteristically very thin and often require considerable amounts of insulin to maintain or increase body weight. However, withdrawal of insulin does not precipitate ketoacidosis. This variety of diabetes was first described by Hugh-Jones in Jamaica[25] and designated by him J Type diabetes. It has subsequently been described in many tropical countries. In India, Tripathy and Kar[26] noted that most patients with this type of diabetes presented between the ages of 15 and 25 years. Although our knowledge of this diabetes variant is still fragmentary, it appears that undernutrition in childhood leads to physiological changes which account for the age of onset and the cardinal features of insulin insensitivity and resistance to ketosis. Adipose tissue is sparse in amount and fat cells do not readily respond to the usual stimuli that provoke breakdown of fat to fatty acids.

Another tropical diabetes variant is otherwise similar to J Type diabetes, but is associated with pancreatic fibrosis and calcification. Although diabetes secondary to pancreatic disease may occur in more affluent societies, it is uncommon and usually occurs in older individuals, especially alcoholic males. The tropical variety was first clearly described in Indonesia by Zuidema.[27] Seven young people with pancreatic calcification were reported of whom six had diabetes. The syndrome of diabetes with pancreatic calcification in the young has subsequently been described in many tropical countries, but it nevertheless is not typical of populations where protein/calorie malnutrition is common in children, so some other factor(s) must be involved. An association has been noted between the prevalence of pancreatic calcification and the consumption of cassava (manioc, manihot, or tapioca).[28]

Cassava contains a cyanogenetic glycoside in the outer integument of tubers and leaves. Cyanide may be released by the action of an enzyme. Cassava consumption has been associated with both goitre and neuropathy.[29] The goitre is caused by a low intake of iodide and high blood levels of thiocyanate, which is formed by cyanide detoxification. Most of the sulphur for thiocyanate formation is derived from sulphur-containing amino acids. McMillan and Geevarghese[30] have suggested that where there is a sufficiency of amino acids (i.e., protein) in the diet, then cassava can produce goitre. Where protein is deficient then cassava might produce pancreatic damage. Some support for this hypothesis comes from studies in Kerala, India, where pancreatic diabetes and goitre are common, but rarely coincide in the same individual.[30] McMillan and Geevarghese also carried out experiments in rats which supported the hypothesis of cyanide + protein deficiency as a cause of pancreatic disorder, although the rats, while developing recurrent hyperglycaemia during chronic cyanide ingestion, did not develop permanent diabetes.

In the absence of demonstrable pancreatic calcification, there is no certain way of distinguishing J Type diabetes and pancreatic diabetes. Nor is it known whether in pancreatic diabetes the diabetes is consequent upon fibrosis/calcification or is a concomitant. It remains possible that severe protein deficiency in infancy and childhood leads to endocrine pancreatic dysfunction which is common to J Type and pancreatic diabetes, with other factors, e.g., cassava consumption, determining the associated exocrine pancreatic pathology.

COMPLICATIONS OF DIABETES[31]

All varieties of diabetes may be complicated by retinopathy, nephropathy and neuropathy. The major determinant of the frequency and severity of such complications is the duration of the diabetes, though individual factors undoubtedly have a role in diminishing or increasing risk. There is little to suggest that nutrition plays any significant part in the genesis of these complications. Diabetics also are at increased risk of atherosclerosis and associated clinical disease, in particular coronary heart disease. This is true even of countries such as Japan, where coronary heart disease has hitherto been infrequent.[32] However, Japanese diabetics are much less at risk than diabetics in most other affluent countries and those living in Japan itself at less risk than emigrants to Hawaii and California.[33] Here nutritional factors may well have a role. The traditional Japanese diet has been low in total and saturated fat and proportionately high in complex carbohydrate (rice). In a comparison of residents of the Hiroshima Prefecture and emigrants or descendents of emigrants from Hiroshima to Hawaii, it was found that while total energy consumption was similar, Hawaiian Japanese consumed about twice as much animal fat and simple carbohydrates and about half the quantity of complex carbohydrates.[34] In an international study comparing vascular disease in diabetics from fourteen populations, major ECG abnormalities (indicating coronary heart disease) were particularly infrequent in diabetics in Hong Kong and Tokyo, whose serum cholesterol levels were also relatively low.[35] It seems very likely that differences in national food habits account for a large part, if not all, of the variation in observed rates of coronary heart disease in diabetics in different populations.

The evolution of dietary therapy in diabetics has been reviewed by Mann.[36] Since the introduction of insulin the major change has been a gradual increase in the proportion of carbohydrate prescribed. More recently, many physicians have employed a proportionately high carbohydrate/low fat diet, some also advocating carbohydrate sources which are rich in vegetable fibre. Such diets have been shown to not worsen or even improve blood glucose control and to lower low density lipoprotein cholesterol levels.[36] Dietary policy nevertheless still varies considerably. In 1971 the Committee on Food and Nutrition of the American Diabetes Association published recommendations which were updated[37] in 1979. The second report was more specific in its recommendations, suggesting, inter alia, that protein intake should account for 12-20% of total energy intake, carbohydrate 50-60%, with the remaining calories from fat. The level of saturated fatty acids should be decreased to less than 10% of total calories and polyunsaturated fatty acids should supply up to 10% of total calories. The committee also recommended that, wherever acceptable, natural foods containing unrefined carbohydrate with fibre should be substituted for highly refined, low fibre carbohydrates. These principles underly the 'prudent' diet used by Mann and his colleagues[24] in the Oxford trial and may well become the new norm for dietary therapy in diabetics. The American group also make the point, possibly the most important of all, that the detailed dietary prescription must always be tailored to the individual patient.

REFERENCES

(1) National Diabetes Data Group, "Classification and diagnosis of diabetes mellitus and other categories of glucose intolerance," *Diabetes* 28, 1039-1057 (1979).

(2) S. Tsuji and M. Wada (Eds.), *Diabetes Mellitus in Asia* (Excerpta Medica, Amsterdam, 1970).

(3) T. Cohen, "Trends in frequency of juvenile diabetes mellitus in Israel," *Israel J. Med. Sci.* 8, 844-45 (1972).

(4) K.M. West, *Epidemiology of Diabetes and its Vascular Lesions* (Elsevier, New York, 1978) 302.

(5) E.P. Joslin, "The prevention of diabetes mellitus," *J. Amer. Med. Assoc.* 76, 79-84 (1921).

(6) K.M. West and J.M. Kalbfleisch, "Glucose tolerance, nutrition, and diabetes in Uruguay, Venezuela, Malaya and East Pakistan," *Diabetes* 15, 9-18 (1966).

(7) K.M. West and J.M. Kalbfleisch, "Diabetes in Central America," *Diabetes* 19, 656-663 (1970).

(8) K.M. West and J.M. Kalbfleisch, "Influence of nutritional factors on prevalence of diabetes," *Diabetes* 20, 99-108 (1971).

(9) R.F. Hamman, P.H. Bennett and M. Miller, "Incidence of diabetes among the Pima Indians," *Advances in Metabolic Disorders* 9, 49-63 (1978).

(10) P. Zimmet and P. Taft, "The high prevalence of diabetes mellitus in Nauru, a Central Pacific island," *Advances in Metabolic Disorders* 9, 255-240 (1978).

(11) J.V. Neel, "Diabetes mellitus: A 'thrifty' genotype rendered detrimental by progress'?" *Amer. J. Hum. Genet.* 14, 353-362 (1962).

(12) H.P. Himsworth, "Diet and the incidence of diabetes," *Clinical Sci.* 2, 117-148 (1935-6).

(13) J. Yudkin, "Dietary fat and dietary sugar in relation to ischaemic heart disease and diabetes," *Lancet* II, 4-5 (1964).

(14) T.L. Cleave, *The Saccharine Disease* (Wright, Bristol, 1974).

(15) A.M. Cohen, "Environmental aspects of diabetes," *Israel J. Med. Sci.* 8, 358-363 (1972).

(16) H. Keen, B.J. Thomas, R.J. Jarrett and J.H. Fuller, "Nutrient intake, adiposity and diabetes," *Brit. Med. J.* 1, 655-658 (1979).

(17) K.M. West, *Epidemiology of Diabetes and its Vascular Complications* (Elsevier, New York, 1978) 248 et seq.

(18) K.M. Hambidge, "Chromium nutrition in man," *Amer. J. Clinical Nutr.* 27, 505-514 (1974).

(19) J.F. Bale Jr., "John Harvey Kellogg MD and the American diet," *University of Michigan Medical Center J.* 41, 56-58 (1975).

(20) H.C. Trowell, "Dietary-fiber hypothesis of the etiology of diabetes mellitus, *Diabetes* 24, 762-765 (1975).

(21) J.W. Andersen and W-JL. Chen, "Plant fiber. Carbohydrate and lipid metabolism," *Amer. J. Clinial Nutr.* 32, 346-363 (1979).

(22) P.A. Crapo, G. Reaven and J. Olefsky, "Postprandial plasma-glucose and plasma-insulin responses to different complex carbohydrates," *Diabetes* 26, 1178-83 (1977).

(23) J.M. Munoz, H.H. Sandstead and R.A. Jacob, "Effects of dietary fiber on glucose tolerance of normal men," *Diabetes* 28, 496-502 (1979).

(24) R.W. Simpson, J.I. Mann, J. Eaton, R.A. Moore, R. Carter and T.D.R. Hockaday, "Improved glucose control in maturity-onset diabetes treated with high carbohydrate-modified fat diet," *Brit. Med. J.* 1, 1753-1756 (1979).

(25) P. Hugh-Jones, "Diabetes in Jamaica," *Lancet* II, 891-897 (1955).

(26) B.B. Tripathy and B.C. Kar, "Possible role of nutrition on the pattern of diabetes in the tropics," in *Diabetes in the Tropics* (Eds. J.C. Patel and N.G. Talwalkar) (Diabetic Association of India, Bombay), 446-452.

(27) P.J. Zuidema, "Calcification and cirrhosis of the pancreas in patients with deficient nutrition," *Documenta de Medicina Geographica et Tropica* 7, 229-251 (1955).

(28) C.S. Pitchumoni, "Pancreas in primary malnutrition disorders," *Amer. J. Clinical Nutr.* 26, 374-379 (1973).

(29) "Chronic cassava toxicity," *Lancet* II, 245-246 (1973).

(30) D.E. McMillan and P.J. Geevarghese, "Dietary cyanide and tropical malnutrition diabetes," *Diabetes Care* 2, 202-208 (1979).

(31) H. Keen and J. Jarrett (Eds.), *Complications of Diabetes* (Arnold, London, 1975).

(32) Y. Goto, S-I. Sato and M. Masuda, "Causes of death in 3151 diabetic autopsy cases," *Tohoku J. Exper. Medic.* 112, 339-353 (1974).

(33) A. Kogan, B.R. Harris, W. Winkelstein, Jr., K.G. Johnson, H. Kato, I.S. Syme, G.G. Rhoads, M.L. Gay, M.Z. Nichaman, H.B. Hamilton and J. Tillotson, "Epidemiologic studies of coronary heart disease and stroke in Japanese men living in Japan, Hawaii and California: demographic, physical, dietary and biochemical characteristics," *J. Chronic Diseases* 27, 345-364 (1974).

(34) R. Kawate, M. Yamakido, Y. Nishimoto, P.H. Bennett, R.F. Hamman and W.C. Knowler, "Diabetes mellitus and its vascular complications in Japanese migrants on the island of Hawaii," *Diabetes Care* 2, 161-170 (1979).

(35) H. Keen and R.J. Jarrett, "The WHO Multinational Study of Vascular Disease in Diabetes: 2. Macrovascular disease prevalence," *Diabetes Care* 2, 187-195 (1979).

(36) J.I. Mann, "Diet and diabetes," *Diabetologia* 18, 89-95 (1980).

(37) Special Report: "Principles of nutrition and dietary recommendations for individuals with diabetes mellitus: 1979. *Diabetes* 28, 1027-1030 (1979).

-10-

Diet and Diabetes

Alan Chait and Edwin L. Bierman

SUMMARY

From the preinsulin era until the present time, dietary management has been considered fundamental in the therapy of the diabetic patient. Despite the emphasis given to dietary management of both insulin-dependent and non-insulin dependent diabetes in textbooks of medicine, recent studies both in the U.S.A. and Britain have shown that most diabetics receive inadequate dietary advice and counselling.[1-3] Recommendations, when given, vary widely, particularly with respect to the composition of the diet. Of those patients that are presented a specific diet, many fail to adhere to recommendations.[1] Against this background of inadequate dietary advice and education on the part of health professionals, and of poor compliance by diabetic patients, it is worth reevaluating the role of the diet in the management of diabetes, with particular emphasis on the potential benefits to be accrued by compliance with a dietary regime.

CONSEQUENCES OF DIABETES THAT MAY BE INFLUENCED BY DIET

Macrovascular Complications

Atherosclerosis has become the major cause of morbidity and mortality among diabetics today, accounting for more than 60% of diabetic deaths in the U.S.A. In diabetics, of both insulin-dependent and non-insulin dependent types, atherosclerotic complications are more severe and occur earlier than in non-diabetics, and in diabetics the relative immunity against the development of atherosclerotic complications seen in non-diabetic females is lost.[4] Multiple risk factors for the development of atherosclerosis have been identified in the population at large; several of these appear to occur more commonly among diabetics. Hyperglycemia, per se, by mechanisms not yet understood, appears to be a major risk factor for the development of atherosclerosis. Both retrospec-

117

tive and prospective studies of cardiovascular risk factors clearly demonstrate that hyperglycemia occurs commonly among subjects who develop coronary artery disease.[4] Conversely, diabetics have a higher incidence of cardiovascular complications than their matched non-diabetic counterparts.[4]

Hypercholesterolemia, which has long been known to be a potent atherosclerosis risk factor, occurs more commonly in the diabetic than in the general population,[5] possibly in part due to the low carbohydrate, high fat diet traditionally prescribed for diabetics for the past few decades. Hypertriglyceridemia, a more controversial cardiovascular risk factor, is a feature of uncontrolled diabetes that tends to correct with improved blood glucose control.[4,6,7] Although not all forms of hypertriglyceridemia predispose to the development of atherosclerosis, hypertriglyceridemia in association with diabetes does appear to.[8,9] Reduced high density lipoprotein (HDL) cholesterol, a recently rediscovered cardiovascular risk factor, occurs commonly in obese non-insulin dependent diabetics and may play a role in the development of early onset atherosclerotic complications.[10]

Hypertension is more prevalent in diabetics than non-diabetic populations[4,11] as is obesity,[4,12] which although not necessarily an independent cardiovascular risk factor, assumes importance because it commonly is associated with hyperlipidemia and hypertension. Insulin itself has been implicated in atherogenesis and has been shown to be an independent risk factor for coronary heart disease in the non-diabetic.[13] Diabetics tend to have high circulating insulin levels, whether in the obese adult diabetic who has hyperinsulinemia as a consequence of obesity, or in the insulin-treated patient due to the inability to regulate precisely the amount of insulin required at any time. Thus, during the 24 hour period, inappropriately high circulating insulin levels may be present for much of the time in patients receiving insulin. In all types of diabetes, arterial wall metabolism might be altered by exposure to high circulating insulin (and lipoprotein) levels.

Although poorly understood at present, it is possible that genetic factors in diabetes, by virtue of an intrinsic defect in cellular metabolism, also could predispose the diabetic to the development of atherosclerosis.

Several of these cardiovascular risk factors can be treated by diet, both in non-diabetic and in diabetics. Thus, any dietary recommendations for diabetic patients should have as a primary goal prevention of atherosclerotic complications or at least delaying or minimizing their occurrence.

Microvascular Complications

The other serious group of diabetic complications consists of the microvascular disorders that result in retinopathy and nephropathy. Diabetic retinopathy is the leading cause of blindness in the U.S.A. today, and nephropathy is the second commonest cause of mortality in diabetics after cardiovascular disease. The role of hyperglycemia and the effect of blood glucose control in the etiology of these complications remains controversial. Many studies, particularly those in diabetic patients, have failed to demonstrate that good diabetic control prevents the onset of these microvascular complications.[14] However, by current criteria, even with excellent blood glucose control using therapeutic regimes that are widely available, many metabolic disturbances persist. With the advent of the new insulin delivery systems, it may for the first time prove feasible to approach normal metabolic homeostasis in diabetics, after which it will be possible to study the effect of good metabolic control on the development of microvascular complications. Despite present day limitation, many studies, both in experimental animals and man, do suggest that persistent hyperglycemia may play a role in the development of both retinopathy and nephropathy. Perhaps the most convincing evidence comes from experimental animal studies in which lesions resembling diabetic glomerulosclerosis develop in untreated diabetic animals, and can be prevented from occurring by insulin-treatment.[15,16]

Definitive answers as to the effect of good blood glucose control on the development of microvascular complications are unlikely to be available for several years. In the meantime, on the basis of the experimental and epidemiological information available, it seems reasonable to aim for blood glucose levels as near the physiological range as is feasible. However, in attempting to normalize diurnal blood glucose levels, caution should be exercised to avoid hypoglycemia, since recurrent hypoglycemic episodes can have serious consequences on cerebral function.

Diabetic Control

Management of diabetes in general, not just with diet, should of course also aim at preventing the short-term consequences of the diabetic state. Hyperglycemia leads to glycosuria, osmotic diuresis and the symptoms of polyuria, polydypsia with short-term complications such as monilial infections. The catabolic state associated with untreated diabetes results in weight loss, weakness and poor resistance to infections. Although correction of these metabolic abnormalities is a primary goal of therapy, any approach to management of the diabetic should reach beyond these short-term objectives and should aim to prevent or at least delay and minimize these more serious and debilitating long-term macrovascular and microvascular complications that eventually occur in diabetics of all types.

Although it is not yet known whether any of these long-term objectives can be accomplished by diet, some metabolic manifestations of diabetes can be influenced by diet. These include reversal of abnormal blood glucose levels, insulin levels, glucose excretion, plasma lipid levels (cholesterol and triglyceride) and body weight. The most interesting and potentially most effective dietary intervention is caloric restriction to effect weight reduction, since this maneuver will result in correction of all the other metabolic abnormalities that can be affected by diet. Thus, weight reduction results in a lowering of plasma glucose levels, elimination of glycosuria and lowering of both plasma cholesterol and triglyceride levels. All of these are of potential value in the prevention of macro- and microvascular complications. Since the vast majority of adult diabetics are overweight,[17] caloric restriction to achieve weight reduction becomes a logical goal and is the single most important aspect of dietary management of overweight diabetic patients. Lean insulin-dependent diabetics on the other hand require sufficient calories for normal growth and development, and in this group, and for those non-insulin dependent diabetics at their ideal weight, the dietary regime recommended should take into consideration both short- and long-term consequences of diabetes.

THE DIABETIC DIET

The nutritional management of diabetes mellitus must take into account the two main clinical types of diabetes, because, although certain aspects of the diets are similar, other aspects differ. Already alluded to is the difference in energy requirements between obese and lean diabetics. The other major consideration is whether or not the diabetic (whether insulin-dependent, i.e., ketosis-prone, or not) is taking insulin, for then the timing of meals becomes a critical consideration in achieving diurnal blood glucose levels near the physiological range, while at the same time avoiding hyperglycemia. Finally, since a prime goal of the diet is prevention of atherosclerosis, a reduced intake of saturated fat and cholesterol should be part of the dietary recommendation.

Energy Balance

From a practical standpoint, dietary therapy in diabetes mellitus should aim first and foremost at providing an appropriate total calorie intake: caloric restriction in the overweight non-insulin dependent diabetic and the presence of adequate calories to maintain normal growth and development in insulin-dependent juvenile type diabetics.

In many obese diabetics, reversal of the impaired glucose tolerance to normal can be achieved simply by weight reduction.[18] In more severe cases, weight reduction often allows the dose of insulin or oral hypoglycemic agents to be lowered or in some cases for their use to be discontinued. In addition, weight reduction and maintenance of a new and lower steady state weight leads to reduction of elevated blood pressure levels, plasma cholesterol and triglyceride, all of which are prominent risk factors for atherosclerosis.[19] Desirable weight for adults can easily be determined from insurance company actuarial tables. The diet prescribed, while restrictive in calories, should be nutritionally adequate and balanced. Within this framework, the composition of the diet is not critical during periods of rapid weight loss. If calories are severely restricted (e.g., less than 1,000 calories/day), vitamin and mineral supplementation to provide minimal daily requirements is advisable, particularly in cases in which prolonged caloric restriction is anticipated. Long-term results of sustaining weight loss are uniformly bad in non-diabetics; more than 90% of patients generally regain their initial weight within 5-10 years after reaching their nadir. For this reason, diabetic patients on weight loss regimens require much encouragement and support with frequent follow-up visits.

The improvement of glucose tolerance associated with weight loss is due to reversal of the insulin resistance that occurs in association with obesity. This insulin resistance at the level of peripheral tissues results in compensatory hypertrophy of the pancreatic islets, and leads to hyperinsulinemia, with high basal plasma insulin levels. Thus diet and not insulin is the logical treatment of choice for those usually uncomplicated mild to moderate obese adult diabetics. In more severe cases, additional therapy, oral agents or insulin, may need to be added in order to treat symptoms associated with hyperglycemia. In such cases, these additional therapies will be much more effective in the presence of calorie restriction, weight loss and reduced insulin resistance. Unfortunately, for many years calorie restriction was believed to be an essential requirement in the diet of all diabetics, a misconception that no doubt led to retardation of normal growth and development of many juvenile insulin-dependent diabetics in the past. In these patients, undernutrition tends to be more of a problem than overnutrition, and sufficient calories are an essential prerequisite for normal growth and development. Young onset non-insulin-dependent diabetes (also referred to as maturity onset diabetes of the young or MODY) should be treated like adult non-insulin-dependent diabetes except that adequate calories should be given during the adolescent growth spurt. However, as in the adult type of diabetic, careful attention should be given to weight, and attempts to prevent obesity should commence at an early age. For the diabetic, insulin- or non-insulin-dependent, at ideal weight, the mainstay of therapy is total calorie control to provide a nutritionally adequate diet for maintenance of weight and avoidance of weight gain with increasing age. Now the composition of the diet becomes important and will be considered both with respect to blood glucose homeostasis and to the prevention of atherosclerotic complications.

Diet Composition

The composition of the diabetic diet, specifically the proportion of total calories to derive from carbohydrate vs fat, remains a controversial area in which opinions have oscillated considerably over the years. Preferences for either high or low carbohydrate diets have dominated thinking at different times in the history of diabetic management. However, a careful review of some of the early studies concerning diet suggests that much of the information that provides the basis for current recommendations of high carbohydrate intake has been known for years. Also, since it was realized that atherosclerotic complications are the major cause of morbidity and mortality in diabetics of all types, and since there is some consensus that a diet low in saturated fat and cholesterol is of value in the prevention of atherosclerosis in the population at large, the pendulum has swung to a diet that emphasizes fat restriction and a relatively high carbohydrate content. This low fat, moderately high carbohydrate diet forms the basis of the new dietary recommendations of the Food and Nutrition Committee of the American Diabetes Association.[20] Although proof of the dietary-fat hypothesis of atherogenesis is lacking, sufficient circumstantial evidence exists to warrant a dietary approach to the prevention of heart disease in the general population.[21] Therefore, it seems entirely reasonable to pursue a similar approach to the prevention of atherosclerosis in diabetic patients, who are clearly at even greater risk of developing atherosclerotic complications. Also, an increase in carbohydrate intake to the levels recommended appears to be beneficial to blood glucose homeostasis.

The low carbohydrate diets in vogue in the 1930's and 1940's traditionally emphasized very high saturated fat intake, which is likely to have contributed to the development of atherosclerotic complications in already prone individuals during that period of time. The high carbohydrate approach fell into relative disfavor and has only reemerged in the last decade or so. Despite dietary recommendations by such bodies as the American Diabetes Association,[20] the use of a high carbohydrate, low-fat diet in diabetes clearly has not yet received worldwide recognition.[2]

The early evidence that high carbohydrate diets are beneficial to blood glucose control are convincing. These studies, pioneered by Himsworth, demonstrated that the higher the amount of carbohydrate in the diet of young non-diabetic volunteers, the better was the glucose tolerance.[22] With severe carbohydrate restriction, glucose tolerance becomes abnormal; these observations form the basis for the recommendation for a carbohydrate intake of at least 300 g daily prior to glucose tolerance testing.

The improved glucose tolerance with high carbohydrate intake was attributed to increased insulin sensitivity resulting from these diets. These observations have been reconfirmed over the years, for example by Anderson[23] and Brunzell[24] in the 1970's. Both groups studied normal subjects under carefully controlled metabolic ward conditions and demonstrated that glucose tolerance was improved by increasing the carbohydrate content of the diet to as high as 80-85% of total calories. Improved glucose tolerance was observed by Brunzell in mild non-insulin dependent diabetics as well, most of the improvement being due to lower fasting plasma glucose levels. Glucose disappearance rates after intravenous insulin improved on the high carbohydrate diets.[23]

The improved glucose tolerance on high carbohydrate diets does not appear to depend on the nature of the carbohydrate since similar changes were observed whether or not sucrose was present as the carbohydrate source.[25] Similar findings were observed in diabetics on treatment with insulin or oral glucose-lowering agents. Fasting plasma glucose and 24 hour urinary glucose was lower in diabetics consuming liquid formula diets in which 85% of calories were provided as carbohydrate than when compared to 40% carbohydrate diets.[26] Only untreated, decompensated diabetics were unable to handle the extra dietary carbohydrate load. Thus, when sufficient insulin is available, either exogenous for diabetics receiving insulin, or endogenous in obese non-insulin dependent diabetics, increasing the carbohydrate content even to fairly extreme levels, improves glucose tolerance. As a result of increased sensitivity, insulin dosage can be reduced substantially without adversely affecting glucose homeostasis.

The studies cited were performed under carefully controlled conditions on a metabolic ward. Although much less is known about the effect of high carbohydrate diets in free-living diabetics, the few studies reported strongly suggest that similar findings pertain under these conditions. Stone and Connor[27] prospectively tested the effect of long-term outpatient high carbohydrate, low fat, low cholesterol diets in insulin-dependent diabetics over a 2 year period. They demonstrated that the experimental diet, containing 20% fat, 64% carbohydrate and 100 mg cholesterol/day, resulted in no change in weight and no increase in insulin requirements, which actually decreased in some patients. There was a highly significant reduction in plasma cholesterol levels and also a reduction in plasma triglyceride when compared to the control diet that contained 42% fat, 41% carbohydrate and 900 mg cholesterol/day. A recently reported study from England showed similar results. Newly diagnosed diabetics were randomly allocated to either a low carbohydrate, high fat or a relatively high carbohydrate, low-fat group. After one year of follow-up, blood glucose levels were similar in the two groups, but plasma cholesterol was lower in the diabetics on the low fat, high carbohydrate diet.[28] Thus, outpatient diets high in carbohydrate and low in fat appear to have no deleterious effect on diabetic control and are perhaps beneficial with regard to hyperlipidemia and the prevention of atherosclerosis to which diabetics are so prone.

Further, high carbohydrate diets do not appear to result in a sustained increase in plasma triglyceride levels. In fact, recent attention to plasma levels throughout the 24 hour period indicate that triglycerides may actually decrease during the day on high carbohydrate diets,[29] while 24 hour glucose levels are not increased.[30]

Hyperlipidemia commonly accompanies diabetes. Hypertriglyceridemia, the most frequent plasma lipid abnormality seen, often reflects the adequacy of diabetic control.[4] Hypercholesterolemia also is more common in diabetes than in the general population. Some diabetic patients also have one of the familial forms of hyperlipidemia. Saturated fat and cholesterol restriction deserve particular emphasis in those diabetics with hyperlipidemia, since the association of hyperlipidemia with diabetes appears to be of particular importance in the predisposition of the diabetic to atherosclerosis.[8,9]

Practical Recommendations

The important dietary concepts that have evolved over the years have been adopted in the recommendations from the Food and Nutrition Committee of the American Diabetes Association published during the last decade.[20] They advise that carbohydrate intake should be increased to 50-60% of total calories in diabetics. Fat should account for approximately 30% of calories and should be divided equally among polyunsaturated, monounsaturated and saturated fats. Increasing the polyunsaturated fatty acid content above this level is not recommended in view of present uncertainties about the long-term effects of a diet rich in these fatty acids. Cholesterol intake should be restricted. In the presence of hypercholesterolemia and hypertriglyceridemia, further fat and cholesterol restriction should be considered. Since simple sugars tend to be rapidly absorbed from the intestinal tract, it is reasonable to try and limit blood glucose fluctuations in more severe diabetics by limiting the use of excess glucose and glucose containing disaccharides (lactose and sucrose). Addition of fiber to the diets of diabetics may significantly lower postprandial blood glucose levels, and limit diurnal blood glucose excursions.[31,32] Dietary fiber comes in many forms and the effect of the specific types on blood glucose homeostasis remains to be clearly defined. However, it is likely that the use of a diet high in food fiber will prove to be beneficial for minimizing postprandial blood glucose excursions.

Another factor that is of utmost importance in minimizing blood glucose fluctuation is the timing of meals in diabetics on insulin. Because the delivery of insulin is not regulated by physiological needs, carbohydrate calorie intake needs to be distributed throughout the day to provide adequate glucose upon which the absorbed insulin can act. From a practical standpoint, diabetic patients on insulin should consume some carbohydrate calories every 3-4 hours during the hours that they are awake. The bedtime snack is of special importance in view of recent reports suggesting that asymptomatic and undiagnosed hypoglycemia is a frequent nocturnal occurrence in patients taking insulin.[33,34] Attention to the timing of meals can lower blood glucose excursions and result in less hypoglycemia in patients on insulin.

Two other considerations that may be important in blood glucose control and in the prevention of macrovascular complications in diabetics are alcohol and exercise.

Epidemiological studies suggest that alcohol, consumed in moderate quantities, may protect against the development of coronary artery disease in the population at large.[35,36] This effect has been attributed to the ability of alcohol to raise circulating levels of high density lipoprotein,[37] a lipoprotein that appears to confer protection from heart disease.[38] Therefore, it seems reasonable that diabetics should be permitted to consume alcohol in limited amounts provided, firstly, that it is within the confines of their caloric allowance, and secondly, that a number of precautions are observed. Sweet alcohol beverages and mixers should be avoided to limit fluctuations in blood glucose levels. Since alcohol can result in hypoglycemia both in non-diabetic and diabetic subjects, symptoms of hypoglycemia after alcohol consumption should not be confused with drunkenness. The hypoglycemic effect of ethanol can usually be prevented by the consumption of alcohol in a mixed meal setting. Finally, attention should be paid to the plasma triglyceride level because some hypertriglyceridemic subjects, including diabetics, are extremely sensitive to the triglyceride raising properties of alcohol.[39] However, in most diabetics, particularly if at ideal body weight, limited alcohol usage may be beneficial to the patient.

Exercise has long been thought to be of value in protecting against heart disease. Recent studies have suggested that this effect, like that of alcohol, may be mediated through elevated high density lipoprotein levels,[40] although plasma triglyceride also tends to fall with exercise, possibly as a result of weight loss. Participation in a regular exercise program may therefore be of benefit in diabetes, particularly in overweight patients. However, some caution is required when vigorous exercise is undertaken by diabetics on insulin, since exercise improves glucose disposal and causes a more rapid release of insulin from subcutaneous depots, thereby predisposing to hypoglycemia. A reduced dose of insulin on days during which vigorous exercise will be undertaken may be of value in preventing hypoglycemia, but most patients prefer rather to increase their carbohydrate consumption in anticipation of the increased need.

These various dietary recommendations should be integrated with a program that is individualized according to the patients' personal needs. Social habits, lifestyle, dietary preferences, cultural and socio-economic factors and psychological make-up all need to be considered when devising a diet for a specific patient. These factors need to be integrated with other aspects of the patient's disease, other therapeutic modalities, complications that might be present and any other coexisting medical conditions. By maintaining flexibility within defined guidelines, compliance with a program, which by necessity needs to be life-long, will hopefully be improved. The basic dietary approach discussed has evolved through better understanding of diabetes, its various subgroups, its natural history and complications. Dietary approaches, like other forms of therapy, will no doubt continue to be modified, as our understanding increases.

REFERENCES

(1) K.M. West, "Diet therapy of diabetes: an analysis of failure," *Ann. Int. Med.* 79, 425-434 (1973).

(2) B. Thomas, A.S. Truswell and A. Brown, "Diabetic diet sheets used in Great Britain. I. Aspects of presentation and content," *Nutrition* 28, 297-312 (1974).

(3) R. Tunbridge and J.H. Wetherill, "Reliability and cost of diabetic diets," *Brit. Med. J.* 2, 78-80 (1970).

(4) E.L. Bierman and J.D. Brunzell, "Atherosclerosis, abnormal lipid metabolism and diabetes," in: *Advances in Modern Nutrition* 2, H.M. Katzen, R.J. Mahler (eds.) (Wiley & Sons, New York, 1978).

(5) M.I. New, T.N. Roberts, E.L. Bierman and G. Reader, "The significance of blood lipid alterations in diabetes mellitus," *Diabetes* 12, 208 (1963).

(6) J.D. Brunzell, D. Porte Jr. and E.L. Bierman, "Reversible abnormalities in postheparin lipolytic activity during the late phase of release in diabetes mellitus," *Metab. Clin. Exp.* 24, 1123-1137 (1975).

(7) B. Lewis, M. Mancini, M. Matlock, A. Chait and T.R. Fraser, "Plasma triglyceride and fatty acid metabolism in diabetes mellitus," *Eur. J. Clin. Invest.* 2, 445-453 (1972).

(8) R.J. Santen, P.W. Willis and S. Fajans, "Atherosclerosis in diabetes mellitus," *Arch. Int. Med.* 130, 833-843 (1972).

(9) R. Kawate, M. Miyanishi, M. Yamakido and Y. Nishimoto, "Preliminary studies of the prevalence and mortality of diabetes mellitus in Japanese in Japan and on the island of Hawaii," *Adv. Metabl. Dis.* 9, 201-224 (1979).

(10) T. Gordon, W.P. Castelli, M.C. Hjortland, W.B. Kannel and T.W. Dawber, "Diabetes blood lipids and the role of obesity in coronary heart disease risk for women. The Framingham Study," *Ann. Int. Med.* 87, 393-397 (1977).

(11) M.J. Garcia, P.M. McNamara, T. Gordon and W.B. Kannel, "Morbidity and mortality in diabetics in the Framingham study: Sixteen year follow-up," *Diabetes* 23, 105-110 (1974).

(12) D.A. Pyke and N.W. Please, "Obesity, parity and diabetes," *J. Endocrinol.* 15, 26 (1957).

(13) R.W. Stout, "Diabetes and atherosclerosis–the role of insulin," *Diabetologia* 16, 141-150 (1979).

(14) J.S. Skyler, "Complications of diabetes mellitus," *Diabetes Care* 2, 499-504 (1979).

(15) J.M. Bloodworth and R.L. Engerman, "Diabetic microangiopathy in the experimentally diabetic dog and its prevention by careful control with insulin," *Diabetes* 22, 190-209 (1973).

(16) P. Rash, "Prevention of diabetic glomerulopathy in streptozotocin diabetic rats by insulin treatment. Glomerular basement membrane thickness," *Diabetologia* 16, 319-324 (1979).

(17) *Joslin's Diabetes Mellitus* 11th ed. A. Marble (ed.) (Lea & Febiger, Philadelphia, 1971).

(18) L.H. Newburgh and J.W. Conn, "A new interpretation of hyperglycemia in obese middle-aged persons," *JAMA* 112, 7-11 (1939).

(19) J. Olefsky, G.M. Reaven and J.W. Farquhar, "Effects of weight reduction on obesity: studies of lipid and carbohydrate metabolism in normal and hyperlipoproteinemic subjects," *J. Clin. Invest.* 53, 64-76 (1974).

(20) Special report from the American Diabetes Association: Principles of nutrition and dietary recommendations for individuals with diabetes mellitus," *Diabetes* 20, 633-634 (1971); *Diabetes* 28, 1027-1030 (1979).

(21) B. Lewis, "Dietary prevention of ischaemic heart disease–a policy for the 1980's, *Brit. Med. J.* 281, 177-180 (1980).

(22) H.P. Himsworth, "The dietetic factor determining the glucose tolerance and sensitivity to insulin of healthy men," *Clin. Sci.* 2, 67-94 (1935).

(23) J.A. Anderson, R.H. Herman and D. Zakim, "Effect of high glucose and high sucrose diets on glucose tolerance of normal men," *Am. J. Clin. Nutr.* 26, 600-607 (1973).

(24) J.D. Brunzell, R.L. Lerner, W.R. Hazzard, D. Porte, Jr. and E.L. Bierman, "Improved glucose tolerance with high carbohydrate feeding in mild diabetes," *N. Engl. J. Med.* 284, 521-524 (1971).

(25) M.G. Dunningan, T. Fyfe, M.T. McKiddie and S.M. Crosbie, "The effects of isocaloric exchange of dietary starch and sucrose on glucose tolerance, plasma insulin and serum lipids in man," *Clin. Sci.* 38, 1-9 (1970).

(26) J.D. Brunzell, R.L. Lerner, D. Porte, Jr. and E.L. Bierman, "Effects of a fat free, high carbohydrate diet on diabetic subjects with fasting hyperglycemia," *Diabetes* 23, 138-142 (1974).

(27) D.B. Stone and W.E. Connor, "The prolonged effects of a low cholesterol, high carbohydrate diet upon the serum lipids in diabetic patients," *Diabetes* 12, 127-132 (1963).

(28) T.D. Hockaday, J.M. Hockaday, J.I. Mann and R.C. Turner, "A prospective comparison of modified fat-high carbohydrate with standard low carbohydrate dietary advice in the treatment of diabetics: A one year follow-up study," *Brit. J. Nutr.* 39, 357-367 (1978).

(29) G. Schlierf, V. Stossberg and W. Reinheimer, "Diurnal patterns of plasma triglycerides and free fatty acids in normal subjects and in patients with endogenous (type IV) hyperlipoproteinemia," *Nutr. Metab.* 13, 80 (1971).

(30) R.W. Simpson, J.I. Mann, J. Eaton, R.A. Moore, R. Carter and T.D.R. Hockaday, "Improved glucose control in maturity-onset diabetes treated with high-carbohydrate modified fat diet," *Brit. Med. J.* 1, 1753 (1979).

(31) J.W. Anderson, W.R. Midgley and B. Wedman, "Fiber and diabetes," *Diabetes Care* 2, 369-379 (1979).

(32) D.A. Jenkins, "Dietary fiber, diabetes and hyperlipidaemia: progress and prospects," *Lancet* II, 1287-1289 (1979).

(33) E.A. Gale and R.B. Tattersall, "Unrecognised nocturnal hypoglycaemia in insulin-treated diabetics," *Lancet* I, 1049-1052 (1979).

(34) C.M. Asplin, T.D. Hockaday, R.F. Smith and R.A. Moore, "Detection of unrecognised nocturnal hypoglycaemia in insulin-treated diabetics," *Brit. Med. J.* 1, 357-360 (1980).

(35) K. Yano, G.G. Rhoads and A. Kagan, "Coffee, alcohol and risk of coronary heart disease among Japanese men living in Hawaii," *N. Engl. J. Med.* 297, 405-409 (1977).

(36) C.H. Henekens, B. Rosner and D.S. Cole, "Daily alcohol consumption and fatal coronary heart disease," *Am. J. Epidemiol.* 107, 196-200 (1978).

(37) J.J. Barboriak, A.J. Anderson and R.G. Hoffman, "Interrelationship between coronary artery occlusion, high density lipoprotein cholesterol and alcohol intake," *J. Lab. Clin. Med.* 94, 348-353 (1979).

(38) A.J. Miller and N.E. Miller, "Plasma high density lipoprotein concentration and development of ischaemic heart disease," *Lancet* I, 16-19 (1975).

(39) A. Chait, M. Mancini, A.W. February and B. Lewis, "Clinical and metabolic study of alcoholic hyperlipidaemia," *Lancet* II, 62-64 (1972).

(40) P.D. Wood, W. Haskell, H. Klein, S. Lewis, M.P. Stein and J.W. Farquhar, "The distribution of plasma lipoproteins in middle-aged male runners," *Metabolism* 25, 1249-1257 (1976).

-11-

Heavy Metals
and Degenerative Diseases

Derek Bryce-Smith

SUMMARY

Aspects of the aetiological roles of trace elements in certain major degenerative diseases are reviewed. With essential elements such as copper and cobalt, disease states may arise from either deficiency or excess, but the toxic heavy metals cadmium, mercury and lead have no known essential functions and play only a spoiler's role. The toxic effects of heavy metals are strongly modulated by other dietary components. The diseases discussed include osteomalacia, cardiovascular disease, Wilson's disease, kidney disease, neurological disorders, stillbirth, and birth malformations.

Man evolved as a species in a natural environment of 92 chemical elements ranging from the lightest hydrogen (atomic number 1) to uranium (92). Only lighter elements seem to have been utilised by nature for essential roles in life processes. 'Heavy metals' is one of those useful but slightly vague terms which are hard to define precisely, but which is usually taken to mean those metals at the 'thick end' of the Periodic Table, of atomic number greater than 48 (Cd) which have no known useful or essential biological function, and which on the contrary have certain chemical properties which cause them to exert a disruptive and/or inhibitory role in essential biochemical processes. Of all these metals' properties, it is their strong affinity for sulphur, e.g., the $-SH$ pendant groups on cysteine units in proteins, which most gives rise to their toxic effects. Lighter elements such as sodium, calcium, and magnesium have relatively little affinity for sulphur groups.

The toxic heavy metals which are now known to be of the greatest relevance to human health and well-being are cadmium (48), lead (82), and mercury (80). It is questionable whether any metals 'heavier' than cadmium have any essential role, although claims have been made for tin (50) and of course we are all familiar with the essentiality of the non-metal iodine (53) for thyroid function. Sometimes one finds such essential trace elements as copper (29) and cobalt (27) included among the 'heavy metals' since both deficiencies and excessive intake of these can cause disease. Thus Wilson's disease results from a rare metabolic disorder which causes the accumulation of copper to toxic levels. Treatment involves either chelation with penicillamine to promote urinary copper excretion, or administration of zinc to act as a copper antagonist.[1]

A rather different example, resulting from human actions, arose from the seemingly harmless use of about 1 ppm of a cobalt compound to stabilise the froth on beer. This actually caused the deaths of over a hundred people worldwide from a cobalt-induced cardiomyopathy. It is my personal opinion that the trouble probably arose not from cobalt alone, but from synergistic interaction between cobalt and the large amounts of alcohol consumed; for larger amounts of cobalt can be given therapeutically in pernicious anaemia without causing damage to the heart.

CADMIUM AND HEALTH

This latter example serves to illustrate two important facts. Firstly, excess of an essential trace element can be pathogenic. Secondly, the toxicity of heavy metals in general is modulated by interactions with other dietary components and with other essential and toxic inessential trace elements; the effect is not therefore accurately predictable from the dose alone. In many cases we do not yet understand the mechanism of this modulation, but in others it involves the tendency of an inessential and toxic trace element such as, say, cadmium to mimic the action of a closely related essential element. For example, cadmium mimics zinc–an element required for the function of over 100 enzymes, including those involved in the biosynthesis of proteins. (I might add that zinc is a micro-nutrient in which Western diets tend to be deficient. Many nutritionists seem to be unaware of this.) Thus zinc deficiency exacerbates the toxicity of cadmium, and on the other hand extra zinc can protect to some degree against cadmium.

Sometimes the interactions are more subtle. Thus selenium can protect against the toxic effects of arsenic, cadmium and mercury, probably through the immobilisation of these toxic elements by formation of strong metal-selenium bonds. Selenium itself is an essential trace element, but is dangerously toxic in excess, probably because it immobilises copper: selenosis is effectively treated by supplying extra copper. Calcium is also antagonistic to lead because lead metabolism mimics that of calcium–so much so that calcium deficiency in children (and/or zinc deficiency) seems able to induce a form of pica for lead paint which has been responsible for many fatal cases of childhood lead poisoning.[2,3] Such children will actually seek out any high lead paint available and ignore that lower in lead.

On the other hand, the antagonism between calcium and cadmium probably does not involve a mimicing phenomenon. It must be remembered that the kidney and liver are the main storage organs for cadmium. Thus it seems more likely that the calcium-cadmium antagonism stems at least partly from a direct toxic action of cadmium on the kidney tubules whereby calcium homeostasis is disturbed. Excessive loss of calcium in urine from this cause can induce serious calcium mobilisation from skeletal stores, leading to osteoporosis. Fatal cases of this condition have occurred among peasants in the Jintsu River region of Japan, where it is termed 'itai-itai' disease. The trouble was traced to rice which had been grown in paddy fields contaminated with cadmium from a mine upstream.

Itai-itai disease almost invariably occurred among multiparous women just past child-bearing age: Figure 1 shows one of the afflicted women.[4,5] The first symptom is the development of increasing pain in joints and muscles, and this pain may eventually become almost unbearable. The victim can decrease in height as much as two feet as the disease progresses, and deformities and numerous microfractures develop in the skeleton with the increasing brittleness due to loss of calcium and phosphate (Figure 2). Many patients died, and others were left permanently deformed. Susceptibility to the effects of cadmium was probably enhanced by two special factors: firstly, depletion of calcium stores by repeated childbirth and a diet not well supplied with calcium, and secondly, the women's practice of shrouding themselves in black clothes while working out of doors in the paddy fields, thereby keeping sunlight from their skins and inhibiting Vitamin-D stimulated absorption of calcium and phosphate from the small intestine. However, recent animal studies have suggested that in addition to effects on calcium metabolism resulting from kidney damage there may also be a toxic effect of cadmium at the cellular level in bone.[5a]

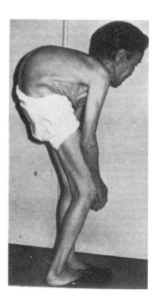

Figure 1. Skeletal deformity in cadmium poisoning ('itai-itai disease')[5]

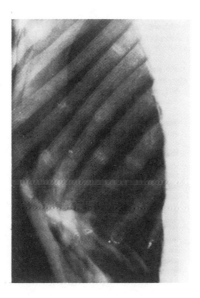

Figure 2. Microfractures in rib-cage: itai-itai disease, Japan[5]

The recent reports of high cadmium levels at Shipham, a village in the Mendip Hills, should serve as a warning that such problems can arise nearer home. No cases of overt disease attributable to cadmium have been reported from Shipham, but proteinuria, an early warning of renal damage, has been found in some individuals. It would be highly desirable to provide zinc and calcium dietary supplements for the inhabitants of such areas, and cigarette smoking, the major individual source of cadmium for smokers, should be very strongly discouraged there. Berkshire County Council is currently concerned about the quite high levels of cadmium now being found in liver and kidney for human consumption. These levels vary and are generally higher than those reported in the 1973 Survey carried out by the Ministry of Agriculture, Fisheries, and Food.[6] It remains to be seen how much of this arises from the frequently cadmium-rich sewage based fertilisers widely distributed to farmers in the Thames Valley.

THE CASE OF LEAD

Lead and arsenic levels in human foodstuffs are currently limited by Statutory Regulations in the U.K. Comparable regulations for cadmium and mercury are urgently required. Blood mercury levels in the U.K. tend to be reassuringly low. Fish is the major dietary source, and in Japan mercury contaminated fish gave rise to the notorious epidemic of poisoning at Minamata, from which many died, and many more have been left permanently afflicted. Most of the mercury in fish is in the specially toxic methylmercury form, CH_3Hg^+. Figure 3 shows that terribly deformed and spastic children were born to mothers who themselves seemed to be unaffected. As Figure 4 shows, the brain is a major target-organ for mercury.[7] I now turn again to cadmium.

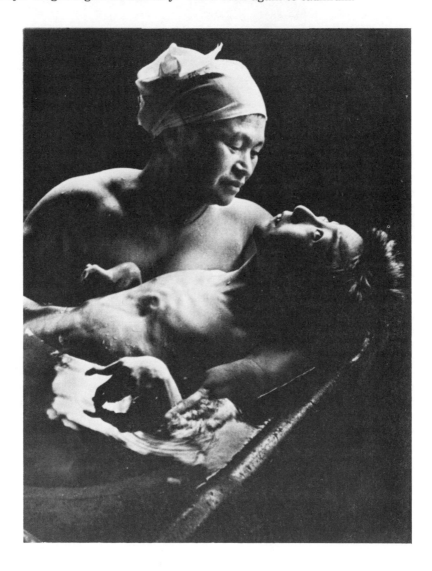

Figure 3. A child damaged by methylmercury in the womb[7]

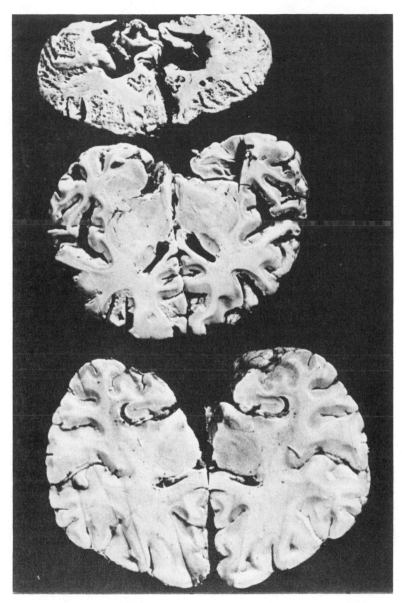

Figure 4. From top: sections of brain from a seven-year-old boy who died after four years of mercury eating away cells; an eight-year-old girl who died after 2 years 9 months; a thirty-year-old man who did not have Minamata Disease[7]

Apart from the well-established kidney damage caused by cadmium, this element is known to induce emphysema, and is a powerful teratogen: see below. There are persistent, though disputed, reports of elevated cadmium levels in hypertension.[5] Such hypertension may well be largely of renal origin, as is the hypertension found at an abnormally high incidence rate among workers in the lead industry. Lead workers are known to suffer abnormally high mortality from renal disease and from non-cardiac hypertensive diseases.[8,9] These findings are suggestive of a connection between cardiovascular disease in the general population and cadmium and/or lead; one is also reminded of the well-known higher cardiovascular mortality rates in soft water than hard water areas. Professor Goldberg and his colleagues have actually reported biochemical and degenerative morphological changes in heart muscle in rats given drinking water at the level of lead found in some Glasgow tapwater (0.5-1.0 ppm) and have suggested that this may be a factor in ischaemic heart disease.[10]

Although a deficiency of such essential elements as calcium and especially magnesium may also be an important part of the 'soft water story',[11,12] lead is also likely to be a factor of importance because of lead induced hypertension and the evidence for a direct toxic effect on heart muscle. In a recent U.K. study by Wibberley and Khere, markedly higher blood lead levels were found in a group of cardiovascular patients than in a comparable group of normotensives (43.9 and 27.9 μg/100 ml respectively). Blood cadmium was also elevated in the patients.[13] This finding is of course consistent with the observations on workers in the lead industry.

It would be extremely interesting to study the effects of chelation therapy using penicillamine or calcium EDTA on a group of hypertensives and a matched control group, but as far as I am aware no studies of this type have been reported. Another approach would be to introduce a dietary regime designed to antagonise lead and cadmium. Such a diet would need to be rich in calcium, phosphate, zinc, manganese, and magnesium, moderately rich in protein and low in fat, fish, and canned food. A general vitamin supplement would be desirable. I am in fact of the opinion that the dietary approach to heavy metal induced diseases would be preferable to chelation therapy. Chelation carries a real though sometimes exaggerated risk of adverse side-effects, especially in older patients, and there can be a loss of essential elements such as copper and zinc together with the toxic metals. Moreover, chelation therapy is not effective in cadmium poisoning, and can even make the condition worse by mobilising body stores of the element.

From my rather limited personal experience, this dietary approach to the treatment of lead intoxication can be remarkably effective, and deserves to be more widely employed. And not only for cardiovascular disease, but also for neurological conditions such as amyotrophic lateral sclerosis and peripheral polyneuropathy where there is evidence for lead as an aetiological factor.[14] Jusic and Sostarko used penicillamine to reduce lead levels in two patients with rapidly progressive spinal amyotrophy, and reported an impressive and sustained improvement.[15] One must not expect success in all cases, and ALS patients do not seem to benefit much from penicillamine.[16] The dietary approach should be tried instead.

Since we are here concerned with 'killer diseases', it would not be appropriate for me to discuss the large body of evidence which now suggests that contemporary body burdens of lead in urban children now regarded as 'normal' are actively pathogenic for mental development and function; for the killing effect there is more on the quality of life than the quantity. I shall accordingly pass over these important aspects and conclude by referring to the evidence for heavy metals as a cause of *fetal* death.

Cadmium, lead, and methylmercury can all cross the placental barrier from the mother, and damage or even kill the developing fetus. Most of the evidence concerning cadmium comes from animal experiments, though not all; and I refer again to Figures 3 and 4 for evidence concerning mercury–the main pathogen in this case was the methylmercury ion, CH_3Hg^+.

Lead of course has long been known as a notorious abortifacient. This property has belatedly been recognised by the U.K. Health and Safety Executive in a Consultative Document published in 1978 which recommended that pregnant women should be prohibited from employment in the lead industry, and that for women of childbearing capacity the maximum blood lead level should be set at *ca.* 40 μg/100 ml, about half the level for all other workers. (There is no evidence that lead at levels of either 40 or 80 μg/100 ml is safe, and much evidence that it is is actively pathogenic; but that is another issue.)

BIRTH ABNORMALITIES

It is known that the incidence of birth abnormalities is much higher in the U.K. than in many other countries. Figure 5 gives the incidence rates for spina bifida deaths. It is known that the incidence of stillbirth and birth malformations is abnormally high in some geographical regions of the U.K., and higher in soft water than hard water areas.[17] My colleagues and I are currently measuring the levels of some 40 elements in tissues from a large number of normal, stillborn, and malformed neonates from several high- and low-risk areas of the U.K. This work will take several years to complete, but I would like to show you the results from a pilot study in which the toxic elements lead and cadmium were measured in bone together with their toxicological antagonists calcium and zinc.[18]

The results for lead and cadmium are shown in Figure 6. The upper limit of normal is set conservatively at 1 μg/g (undried weight basis). It will be seen that 80% of stillbirth lead levels were in excess of this, range 0.1-24.2 μg/g, and 45% of the cadmium levels, range 0.1-31.5 μg/g. Lead and cadmium in individual samples were weakly correlated (r = 0.24). The mean lead and cadmium levels in the stillbirths were some 5-10 times higher than normal. It is also interesting that the levels of all the metals, including calcium and zinc, covered very wide ranges (Figure 7). Many, though by no means all, of these cases must be regarded as having been seriously deficient in one or both of the essential nutrients calcium and zinc. As I mentioned earlier, such deficiencies would tend to exacerbate the fetotoxic effects of the lead and cadmium present in these babies. Support for the idea that lead can be a factor in birth abnormalities has since come from a study by Professor Wibberley and his colleagues at the University of Aston of lead levels in placentae from normal, malformed, and stillborn infants: the levels in placentae from normal births were the lowest.[19] I should mention that the fetus can be harmed not only through the mother, but also through the father as a result of a toxic effect of lead on sperm.[20-22]

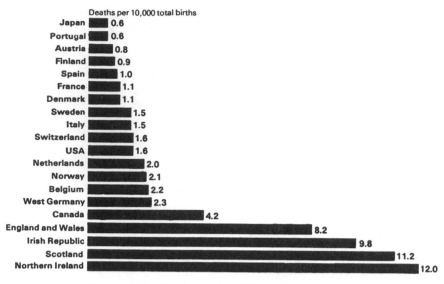

Figure 5. Deaths from spina bifida in first year, 1973

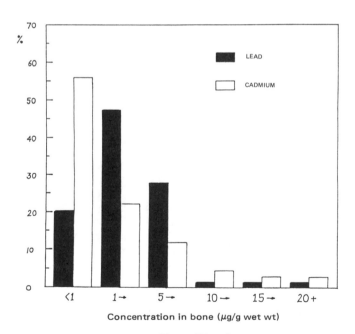

Figure 6. Lead and cadmium in stillbirths

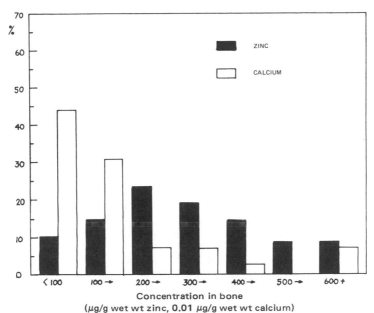

Concentration in bone
(μg/g wet wt zinc, 0.01 μg/g wet wt calcium)

Figure 7. Zinc and calcium in stillbirths

I have not discussed the possible role of heavy metals in such conditions as cancer and multiple sclerosis. There certainly is evidence for at least a supporting role for trace elements in both these multifactorial diseases. It is not well enough known that workers in the lead industry suffer an abnormally high incidence of cancer.[9] But I reserve further comment on these matters for a later occasion. I suggest however it is already apparent from the findings I have summarised that we ought to be paying much more serious attention than we now do to the role of toxic heavy metals as important determinants of the human condition, not just from the cradle to the grave, but rather from the moment of conception; and indeed, even earlier.

REFERENCES

(1) T.V. Hoogenraod, C.J.A. Vanden Hamer, R. Koevoct and E.G.W.M. de Ruyter Korver, "Oral Zinc in Wilson's Disease," *Lancet* II, 1262 (1978); M. Abdulla, "Copper levels after oral zinc," *Lancet* I, 616 (1979).

(2) N.E. Johnson and K. Tenuta, "Diets and Lead Blood Levels of Children Who Practice Pica," *Envir. Res.* 18, 369 (1979).

(3) K.M. Hambidge and A. Silverman, "Pica with Rapid Improvement after Dietary Zinc Supplementation," *Arch. Dis. Childhood* 48, 567 (1973).

(4) I. Murata, T. Horino, Y. Saeki and S. Nakagawa, "Cadmium enteropathy, Renal osteomalacia ('Itai-itai' disease) in Japan," *Bull. Soc. Int. Chin.* 1, 34 (1970).

(5) L. Friberg, M. Piscator and G. Nordberg, *Cadmium in the Environment* (CRC Press, Cleveland, Ohio, 1971) 111.

(5a) C. Anderson and K.D. Danglchuk, "Effect of Cadmium on the Haversian Remodeling System in Dogs," *Calcif. Tissue Int.* 27, 121 (1979).

(6) Anon, "Survey of Cadmium in Food," Ministry of Agriculture, Fisheries, and Food (H.M. Stationery Office, London, 1973).

(7) Figures 3 and 4 are from W.E. Smith and A.M. Smith, *Minamata* (Chatto and Windus, London, 1975).

(8) W.C. Cooper and W.R. Gaffey, "Health Study of Lead Workers," *J. Occup. Med.* 17, 100 (1975); *idem.* Report LH-157 (ILZRO, New York, 1974).

(9) H.K. Kang, P. Infante and J.S. Carra, "Occupational Lead Exposure and Cancer," *Science* 207, 935 (1980).

(10) M.R. Moore, P.A. Meredith, A. Goldberg, K.E. Carr, P.G. Toner, and T.D.V. Lawrie, "Cardiac Effects of Lead in Drinking Water of Rats," *Clin. Sci. Mol. Med.* 49, 337 (1975), *cf.* A.D. Beattie *et al., Br. Med. J.,* 1972, 2, 488, 491.

(11) Anon., "Water quality, Trace Elements, and Cardiovascular Disease," *WHO Chronicle* 27, 534 (1973).

(12) T.W. Anderson, L.C. Neri, G.B. Schreiber, F.D.F. Talbot and A. Zdrojewski, "Ischaemic Heart Disease, Water Hardness, and Myocardial Magnesium" *C.M.A Journal* 113, 199 (1975).

(13) D.G. Wibberley and A.K. Khere, Results presented at a Symposium on Lead, University of Aston, Birmingham (10th July, 1979).

(14) B. Melgaard, J. Clausen and S.C. Rastogi, "Heavy Metal Levels and δ-Aminolaevulinic Acid Dehydrase Levels in Peripheral Polyneuropathy," *Acta Neurol. Scandinav.* 53, 291 (1976).

(15) A Jusic and M. Sostarko, "Penicillamine in Spinal Amyotrophy," *Lancet* II, 1034 (1977).

(16) M.G. Bousser and M. Malier, "Penicillamine in Amyotrophic Lateral Sclerosis," *Lancet* I, 168 (1979); A.O. House, R.J. Abbot, D.L.W. Davidson, I.T. Ferguson, and J.A.R. Leuman, *Br. Med. J.* 2, 1684 (1978).

(17) M. Wynn and A. Wynn, *Prevention of Handicap and the Health of Women* (Routledge and Kegan Paul, London, 1979).

(18) D. Bryce-Smith, R.R. Deshpande, J. Hughes and H.A. Waldron, "Lead and Cadmium Levels in Stillbirths," *Lancet* I, 1159 (1977).

(19) D.G. Wibberley, A.K. Khere, J.H. Edwards and D.I. Rushton, "Lead Levels in Human Placentae from Normal and Malformed Births," *J. Med. Genetics* 14, 339 (1977).

(20) I. Lancranjan, H.I. Popescu, O. Gavanescu, I. Klepsch and M. Serbanescu, "Reproductive Ability of Workmen Occupationally Exposed to Lead," *Arch. Environ. Hlth.* 30, 396 (1975).

(21) R. Der, Z. Fahim, M. Yousef and M. Fahim, "Synergistic Interaction of Lead and Cadmium on Reproduction and Metabolism of Male Rats," *Res. Comm. in Chem. Path. and Pharmacol.* 14, 689 (1976).

(22) M.S. Fahim, Z. Fahim and D.G. Hall, "Effects of Subtoxic Lead Levels on Pregnant Women," *Res. Comm. in Chem. Path. and Pharmacol.* 13, 309 (1976).

12

The Role of Mycotoxins in Certain Idiopathic Disorders and Tumours in Animals and Man

Regina Schoental

SUMMARY

A number of mycotoxins produced by the common microfungi belonging to the *Aspergillus, Penicillium, Fusarium* and certain other species, can induce in experimental animals various acute, chronic, teratogenic and carcinogenic effects. Such mycotoxins (which include aflatoxin B_1, ochratoxin A, the trichothecene, T-2 toxin and the oestrogenic resorcylic acid macro-lactones, zearalenone and zearalenol) are sporadically present in significant concentrations in livestock feeds and in human foods and drinks, and have to be considered as important factors in the aetiology of the respective idiopathic, acute and chronic disorders, fetal defects, and tumours of animals and man.

Mycotoxins, as the name implies are toxic or otherwise noxious substances produced as secondary metabolites by moulds, under specific environmental conditions. The production of a particular mycotoxin depends not only on the strain and species of the microorganism, and the type of substrate, but also on the oxygen tension, temperature, humidity, and the period of growth.[1]

More than 100,000 species of moulds are known, many are almost ubiquitous, especially in the soil. They will grow on any organic matter, and often contaminate agricultural products. Fortunately, not all are toxigenic.[2]

AFLATOXINS

The known toxigenic microfungi have been isolated from mouldy grains which caused livestock disorders and include *Alternaria, Aspergillus, Penicillium* and *Fusarium* species.[1-3] The natural occurrence of mycotoxins in foods and feeds has been reported from various countries.[1-8] High levels of mycotoxins have usually been connected with outbreaks of illness, death, or reproductive disorders in livestock: economic considerations led then to the investigation of causes of such outbreaks, to the isolation of the toxigenic organisms and to the identification of the toxic agents. A number of mycotoxins are carcinogenic;[9,10] these include the hepatotoxic aflatoxins,[11] the nephrotoxic ochratoxins,[12-14] the irritant and gastrotoxic trichothecenes,[15,16] and the oestrogenic zearalenone. [17,18] Aflatoxins were among the first mycotoxins to be recognised as potential economic and health hazards, and have been widely studied. Their intense fluorescence facilitates their identification; hence their popularity with the researchers. As aflatoxins are effective carcinogens in the rat (and many other animal species), inducing various liver and certain other tumours with doses corresponding to a few mg/kg, aflatoxins became the favourite model substances in studies of the mechanism of hepatotoxicity, carcinogenesis, etc.

However, contamination of foodstuffs with aflatoxins occurs mainly in the tropics; they are optimally produced at temperatures between 20-30°C. The Western countries have now specifications that imported feedstuffs (or foods) must not contain more than about 20 ppb of aflatoxin B_1 (Figure 1). The risk to human health from aflatoxins in Great Britain and other Western countries is not serious; this is borne out by the fact that liver cancer represents less than 1% of all cancers in the colder parts of the world.

Moreover, the human liver disorders and liver tumours in the tropics probably have a multifactorial aetiology.[18]

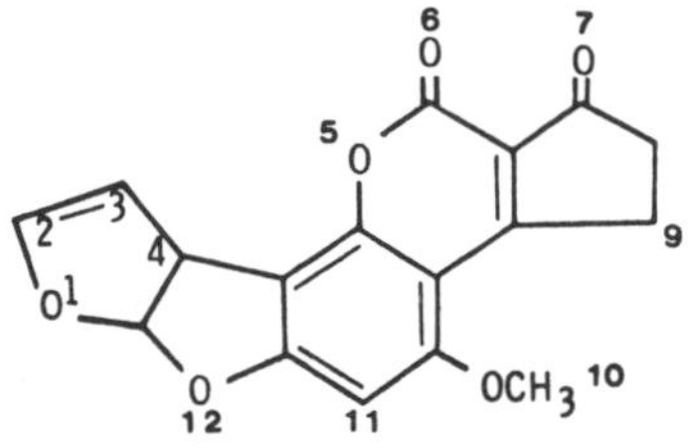

Figure 1. Aflatoxin B_1

OTHER MYCOTOXINS

In contrast to the aflatoxins, contamination of agricultural products by ochratoxin A (Figure 2), trichothecenes [especially T-2 toxin (Figure 3)] and zearalenone occurs often at temperatures below 20°C and high humidity, the conditions which frequently obtain in the parts of the world where epidemiological studies have found high incidence of tumours, nephropathies, gastrointestinal and sex organ disorders, which these mycotoxins, respectively can produce in experimental animals.

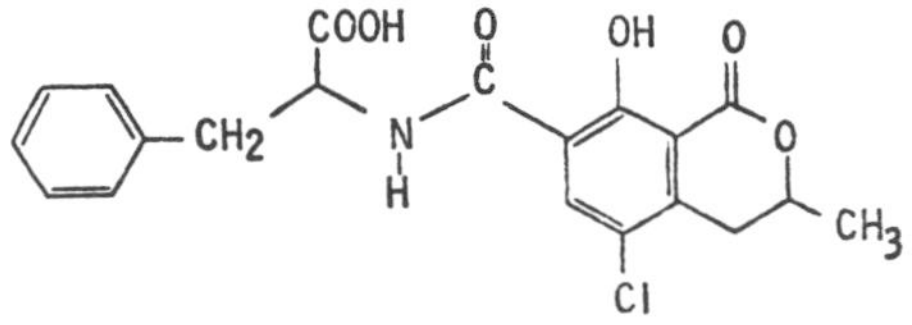

Figure 2. Ochratoxin A

T - 2 Toxin: $R^1 = H$; $R^2 = R^3 = CH_3CO$; $R^4 = (CH_3)_2 CHCH_2CO$

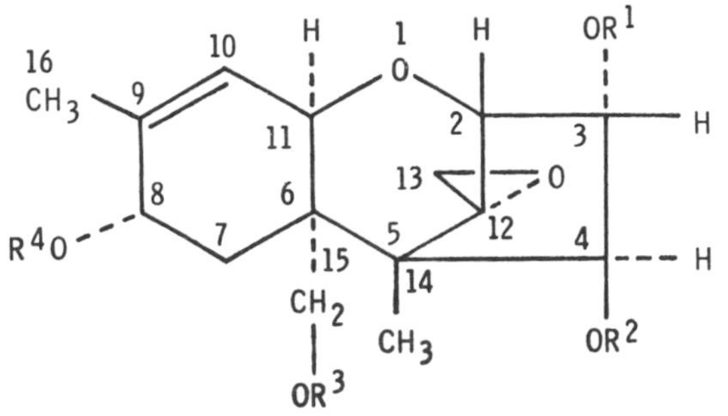

Figure 3. T-2 Toxin

Ochratoxin A (Figure 2) is nephrotoxic[13] and possibly carcinogenic.[14] It has been the subject of detailed studies in Denmark and Sweden in relation to pig nephropathies; in Denmark the levels up to 27 mg/kg (27,000 ppb) have been reported in barley, oats and wheat, and similar levels have been encountered also in Canada.[13] In Denmark, the Agricultural Board issued instructions in 1978, that if at slaughter the pig's kidneys contain more than 10 μg/g (10 mg/kg) of ochratoxin A, the whole carcass of the pig is to be condemned. There appears to be a correlation between the content of ochratoxin A in the kidneys and its blood concentration (50 μg/ml in blood corresponds approximately to 10 μg/g in the kidney).[19] Ochratoxin A may be involved in Balkan nephropathies and kidney tumours. It is teratogenic in experimental animals.[20]

A single or a few doses given at mid-pregnancy can induce foetal abnormalities. The type of defect depends on the day of gestation at the time of transplacental exposure and on the stage of organogenesis, which vary in different animal species.

Ochratoxin A produces a great variety of fetal abnormalities, and indicates how timing of exposure is crucial for the induction of the particular lesions.

The occurrence of neonatal abnormalities and of tumours in man has been known since antiquity. Major developmental anomalies among new-born infants account for 6-7% of all live births; many more are resorbed or aborted Abnormalities not recognisable at birth may become apparent later in life, as intellectual deficiencies, sexual deviations or tumours, which in their majority are due to environmental factors; as such they should be preventable. The lack of preventive measures which could reduce the incidence of many of such incurable disorders is due to the fact that the critical causative agents have not been recognised. Among the critical factors, mycotoxins, including those produced by *Fusarium* species, deserve serious consideration. Many *Fusarium* species produce the estrogenic zearalenone,[17,21] some produce the toxic and irritant trichothecenes,[15] some can produce both these types of metabolites.[5]

Fusarium **FUNGUS**

Fusarium [F. graminearum (Gibberella zeae)] is a common field microfungus which contaminates maize and other cereals. It produces oestrogenic substances, known as zearalenone, 2,4-dihydroxy-6-(10'-hydroxy-6'-oxo-1-undecenyl)benzoic acid-μ-lactone; and zearalenol, 2,4-dihydroxy-6-(6',10'-dihydroxy-1-undecenyl)-benzoic acid-μ-lactone (Figure 4).[17] Zearalenol, like other oestrogenic substances, whether the physiological hormone oestradiol, or the synthetic diethylstilboes-trol, binds to the same receptors and affects the same target organs. The biologi-cal action of oestrogenic compounds depends on the presence (or on the formation in the body) of the two hydroxy-groups at the distance of about 11 Å, in their molecules. Cereals harvested during wet and cold weather can contain (up to 140 mg/kg of) zearalenone.[21] When included in livestock fodder they produce oestrogenism and vulvovaginitis in pigs, abortions, sterility in cattle, etc. Zearalenone in doses of 5-10 mg/kg body weight given to pregnant rats induced significant teratogenic effects in the offspring.[22] The toxicity of zearalenone is very low, but it acts insidiously. High doses would be expected to have similar deleterious teratogenic and carcinogenic effects on the target organs as have other oestrogenic agents in humans and animals.[23-25]

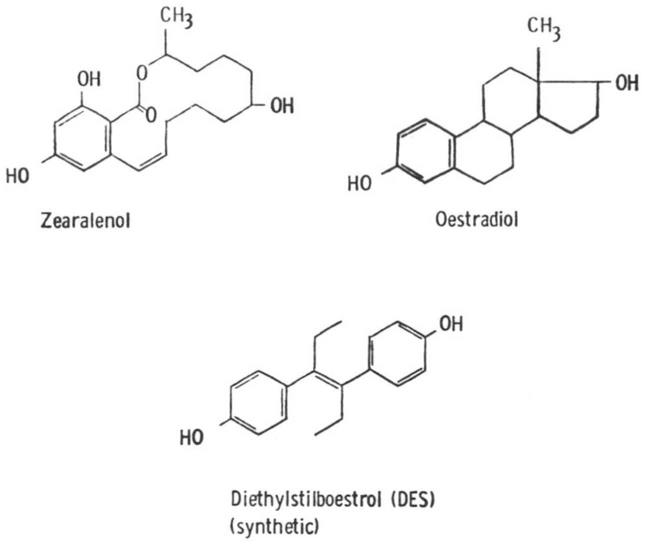

Zearalenol

Oestradiol

Diethylstilboestrol (DES)
(synthetic)

Figure 4. Oestrogenic Compounds

Certain *Fusarium* species can also produce other, more toxic metabolites, which are tetracyclic sesquiterpenes, known as trichothecenes (because the first compound of this structure has been isolated from *Trichothecium* species). Among the three dozen or so trichothecenes already known, one of the most toxic is T-2 toxin.[15,26] Its structure is shown in the figure (Figure 3). The spiro-epoxy ring, the double bond at C(9,10) and at least some of its ester groups are relevant for the biological activity. T-2 toxin was involved in several outbreaks of fatal diseases in man and in animals (some examples of which are sum-marised in Table I).

Table I: Outbreaks of Lethal T-2 Mycotoxicoses in Man and Livestock

Year	Locality	Species	Material Containing T-2	Disorder
1942–3	Orenberg (USSR)	Humans	Bread from over-wintered grain	Alimentary toxic aleukia (ATA)
1970	Wisconsin (USA)	Cows	Mouldy corn fodder	Haemorrhagic diathesis
1970	Hokkaido (Japan)	Horses	Mouldy bean-hulls fodder	Akakabi-byo (*Fusarium* blight)
1976–7	Scotland (GB)	Dairy cows	Mouldy brewers' grains in fodder	Haemorrhagic diathesis
1965–6	Quebec (Canada) USA Belgium	Humans	Beer	Cobalt-beer cardio-myopathy

The most disastrous was the outbreak of a disease known as alimentary toxic aleukia which occurred in Russia, during the Second World War.[27] More than 100,000 people are believed to have died from this disease, which was characterised by the depletion of white corpuscles in the blood, lowered immunity and sore throat. The people died within a few weeks, after having consumed bread made from grain, which unharvested due to war conditions, remained in the field over the winter, became mouldy and contaminated by various microfungi including the toxigenic *Fusarium poae* and *F. sporotrichioides*.

Outbreaks of haemorrhagic disease after consuming mouldy feeds occurred among cattle in the U.S.A.,[4] among horses in Japan[28] and also in Scotland and elsewhere. Nine cows died out of 115 in a dairy herd in Ayrshire in 1977; included in their feeds were mouldy brewers grains which contained T-2 toxin.[29]

An outbreak of cardiomyopathy, which killed at least 40 people in Quebec among heavy beer drinkers[30] and also beer drinkers in the U.S.A. and Belgium during 1967,[31] was probably caused by mouldy grain used for brewing.[32]

T-2 toxin can produce acute and chronic lesions in experimental animals similar to those observed in these outbreaks of human and animal disorders. T-2 toxin does not require activation by liver enzymes, does not damage the liver, and would be expected to similarly affect various species of animals. In long term studies, T-2 toxin induced in rats severe cardiovascular lesions and tumours of the digestive tract and of the brain.[16] T-2 toxin is teratogenic when given to mice on the 10th day of pregnancy, and induced foetal malformations, with doses of 1 or 1.5 mg/kg.[33] T-2 toxin may be involved in the intractable aetiology of human cardiovascular diseases,[34] cancer and neonatal abnormalities. Levels of T-2 toxin exceeding 2 mg/kg have occasionally been reported in grain, especially in Canada, and in the U.S.A.[4] As yet, no quantitative data have been published about the natural occurrence of *Fusarium* mycotoxins in Britain. However, the available evidence indicates that the *Fusarium* mycotoxins may play significant aetiological roles in several disorders (Table II) believed to be "spontaneous", such as reproductive disorders, abortions, foetal anomalies or foetal death, as well as indigestion, cardiovascular diseases and various tumours; they may have been involved in pellagra.[35,36]

Table II: Possible Invovlement of *Fusarium* Mycotoxins
in Certain Disorders and Tumours of Unknown Aetiology

Disorders and Tumours	T-2 Toxin	Zearalenone
1. Abortion	+	+
2: Foetal abnormalities	+	+
3. Sterility, hyperfertility	+	+
4. Sex organ disorders (M & F) and tumours	+	+
5. Cardiovascular disorders	+	?
6. Blood disorders (ATA) leukaemias, lymphomas	+	
7. Decreased immunity, infections ("septic angina")	+	
8. Indigestion, ulcers and tumours of the digestive tract	+	
9. Neurological disorders and brain tumours	+	
10. Diabetes (?), pancreatic tumours	+	

Mycotoxins may be present not only in visibly mouldy products, but also in foodstuffs derived from livestock consuming mouldy fodder (milk, meat, eggs, etc.)[37,38] in alcoholic beverages,[32] tomato[39] and other fruit juices, etc. The possible ill effects, acute or chronic, which may be the result of sporadic ingestion of mycotoxin contaminated foods and drinks remain to be investigated.

It may be significant that one of the trichothecene mycotoxins is known as vomitoxin, or as "feed refusal factor". It has been isolated from feeds, which pigs refused to consume, and identified as 3,7,15-trihydroxy-12,13-epoxytrichothec-9-en-8-one.[40] This compound may be responsible for the vomiting that sometimes follows heavy beer drinking. The tradition in ancient Greece, required that men should abstain from alcoholic drinks before the wedding. This custom, so different from the present day "stag parties", was sound and worth adopting. Alcoholic mothers have been recognised to present risk to their offspring who may develop the "foetal alcohol syndrome".[41,42] The effects on the offspring of fathers indulging in alcoholic sprees, have still to be investigated.

The *Fusarium* mycotoxins, seem to be very important as health hazards in the British Isles, Northern Europe, Canada, U.S.A., etc. Of other mycotoxins already known to have caused ill effects in humans, when present in food, (or used in chemotherapy) mention has to be made of metabolites of ergot *(Claviceps purpurea)* growing on rye which used to be responsible for outbreaks of "St. Anthony's fire" in many countries in Europe; an outbreak occurred in France as recently as in the 1950's.[43,44] In Japan an outbreak of liver disease followed the consumption of yellow rice, imported after the last war from Burma; this was traced to luteoskyrin, and cyclochlorotine, the secondary metabolites of *P. islandicum*.[45]

The study mycotoxins as etiological factors of human and animal disorders is still in its infancy–though they must have affected man and beast as long as life has existed on earth.

Prevention of mycotoxin-contamination of agricultural products is of major importance, economic and humanitarian; it is desirable to develop preventive measures other than fungicides;[46] some of the latter may be no less harmful than the mycotoxins, which they are meant to control. Mycotoxins are immunosuppressive and may play a role in bacterial and viral infections.[47,48]

Appropriate drying and storing of cereals harvested during rainy weather, though expensive, is essential. The recorded outbreaks of mycotoxicoses, whether in man or animals, occur after unusually servere weather conditions.

Under such conditions, the presence of significant amounts of oestrogenic metabolites of *Fusarium* spp. in food, when unrecognised, could confound the effects of therapy of hormone-dependent tumours of the breast and of certain other organs, and result in unexplained lack of response to ovariectomy, or to other hormonal treatments.

REFERENCES

(1) C. Moreau, *Moulds, Toxins and Food*, Translated and Edited by M.O. Moss (John Wiley & Sons, New York, 1979).

(2) C.M. Christensen, *Molds, Mushrooms and Mycotoxins* (Univ. Minnesota Press, Minneapolis, 1975).

(3) L. Stoloff, "Occurrence of mycotoxins in foods and feeds", pp. 23-50 in J.V. Rodricks (Ed.) *Mycotoxins and Other Fungal Related Food Problems,* Advances in Chemistry Series, No. 149 (Amer. Chem. Soc., Washington, DC, 1976).

(4) I.C. Hsu, E.B. Smalley, F.M. Strong and W.E. Ribelin, "Identification of T-2 toxin in moldy corn associated with a lethal toxicosis in cattle," *Appl. Microbiol.* 24, 684-690 (1972).

(5) C.J. Mirocha, S.V. Pathre, B. Schauerhamer and C.M. Christensen, "Natural occurrence of *Fusarium* toxins in feedstuffs," *Appl. Enviro. Microbiol.* 32, 553-556 (1976).

(6) P.M. Scott, "Mycotoxins in feeds and ingredients and their origin," *J. Food Protection* 41, 385-398 (1978).

(7) I.F.H. Purchase (Ed.), *Mycotoxins* (Elsevier Sci. Publ., Amsterdam, 1974).

(8) O.L. Shotwell, C.W. Hesseltine, E.E. Vandegraft, and M.L. Goulden, "Survey of corn from different regions for aflatoxin, ochratoxin and zearalenone," *Cereal Sci. Today* 16, 266-273 (1971).

(9) R. Schoental, "Carcinogens in plants and microorganisms," in *Chemical Carcinogens* (Ed. C.E. Searle) (Am. Chem. Soc. Mongr. 173, Washington, 1976) 626-689.

(10) M. Enomoto, "Carcinogenicity of Mycotoxins" inK. Uraguchi and M. Yamazaki (Eds.), *Toxicology, Biochemistry and Pathology of Mycotoxins* (A Halsted Press Book, John Wiley & Sons, New York London, 1978) 239-362.

(11) R.W. Detroy, E.B. Lillehoj and A. Ciegler, "Aflatoxin and related compounds," in S. Kadis, A. Ciegler and S.J. Ayl (Eds.), *Fungal Toxins* (6, 1971) 4-178.

(12) S. Nesheim, "The ochratoxins and other related compounds," in J.W. Rodrick (Ed.) in *Mycotoxins and Other Fungal Related Food Problems* (Am. Chem. Soc. Adv. Chem. Series No. 149, 1976), 276-295.

(13) P. Krogh, "Causal association of mycotoxic nephropathy, *Acta Path. Microbial Scand. Suppl.* 269, 5-28 (1978).

(14) M. Kanisawa and S. Suzuki, "Induction of renal and hepatic tumors in mice by ochratoxin A, a mycotoxin," *Gann* 69, 599-600 (1978).

(15) J.R. Bamburg and F.M. Strong, "12,13-Epoxytrichothecenes" in *Microbial Toxins,* S. Kadis, A. Ciegler and S.J. Ayl (Eds.) (Vol. 7, 1971), 207-292.

(16) R. Schoental, A.Z. Joffe and B. Yagen, "Cardiovascular lesions and various tumours found in rats given T-2 toxin, a trichothecene metabolite of *Fusarium* species," *Cancer Res.* 39, 2179-2189 (1979).

(17) C.J. Mirocha, S.V. Pathre and C.M. Christensen, "Zearalenone" in *Mycotoxins in Human and Animal Health,* J.V. Rodricks, C.W. Hesseltine and M.A. Mehlman (Eds.) (Park Forest South, Ill. Pathotox Publishers Inc., 1977), 345-364.

(18) R. Schoental, "Mycotoxins" in *Dietary Influences on Cancer: Traditional and Modern,* R. Schoental and T.A. Connors (Eds.) (C.R.P. Press Inc., In Press).

(19) K. Hult, E. Hökby, S. Gatenbeck and L. Rutqvist, "Ochratoxin A blood from slaughter pigs in Sweden: use in evaluation of toxin content of consumed feed," *Appl. Envir. Microbiol.* 39 828-830 (1980).

(20) A.W. Hayes, "Mycotoxin teratogenicity" in *Toxins, Animal Plant and Microbial,* P. Rosenberg (Ed.), *Toxicon,* 17, Suppl 1 (Pergamon Press, Oxford, 1978), 739-758.

(21) J.C. Sutton, W. Baliko and H.S. Funnell, "Relation of weather variables to incidence of zearalenone in corn in Southern Ontario," *Canad. J. Plant Sci.* 60, 149-155 (1980).

(22) J.A. Ruddick, P.M. Scott and J. Harwig, "Teratological evaluation of zearalenone administered orally to the rat," *Bull. Environ. Contamin. & Toxicol.* 15, 678-681 (1976).

(23) International Agency Research on Cancer, "Evaluation of the Carcinogenic Risk of Chemicals to Humans," *Sex Hormones (II) I.A.R.C. Monographs* 21 (1979).

(24) M.B. Lipsett, "Interaction of drugs, hormones and nutrition in the causes of cancer," *Cancer* 43, 1967-1981 (1979).

(25) F.J.C. Roe, "Carcinogenicity studies in animals relevant to the use of anabolic agents in animal production" in *Anabolic Agents in Animal Production,* F.C.Lu and Y. Rendel (Eds.) (G. Thieme Publ., Stuttgart, 1976).

(26) Y. Ueno, "Trichothecenes: Overview address" in *Mycotoxins in Human and Animal Health* (Pathotox Publ. Inc., Forest Park South, Ill., 1977), 189-207.

(27) A.Z. Joffe, "*Fusarium poae* and *F. sporotrichioides* as principal causal agents of alimentary toxic aleukia" in *Mycotoxic Fungi, Mycotoxins, Mycotoxicoses: An Encyclopedic Handook,* T.D. Wyllie and L.G. Morehouse (Eds.) (Marcel Dekker, New York, 1978), 21-86.

(28) Y. Ueno, K. Ishii, K. Sakai, S. Kanaeda, H. Tsunoda, T. Tanaka and M. Enomoto, "Toxicological approaches to the metabolites of *Fusaria*. IV. Microbial survey on 'Bean-Hulls Poisoning of Horses,' with the isolation of trichothecenes, neosolaniol and T-2 toxin of *Fusarium solani* M-1-1," *Jap. J. Exp. Med.* 42, 187-203 (1972).

(29) L. Petrie, J. Robb and A.F. Stewart, "The identification of T-2 toxin and its association with haemorrhagic syndrome in cattle," *Vet. Rec.* 101, 326 (1977).

(30) Y.L. Morin and P. Daniel, "Quebec beer-drinkers cardiomyopathy: Etiological considerations," *Canada. Med. Assoc. J.* 97, 926-928 (1967).

(31) C.S. Alexander, "Cobalt-beer Cardiomyopathy. A Clinical Pathological Study in Twenty-eight Cases," *Am. J. Med.* 53, 395-417 (1972).

(32) R. Schoental, "Disorders and tumors associated with alcoholic drinks–and mycotoxins," *Nutrition and Cancer* 2(2), 88-92 (1980).

(33) G.K. Stanford, R.D. Hood and A.W. Hayes, "Effect of prenatal administration of T-2 toxin to mice," *Res. Commun. Pathol. Pharmacol.* 10, 743-6 (1975).

(34) W.A. Krehl, "The nutritional epidemiology of cardiovascular disease," *Ann. N.Y. Acad. Sci.* 300, 335-359 (1977).

(35) R. Schoental, "Pellagra and *Fusarium* mycotoxins," *Intern. J. Environ. Studies* 13, 327-328 (1979).

(36) R. Schoental, "Mouldy grain and the aetiology of pellagra. The role of toxic metabolites of *Fusarium*," *Biochem. Soc. Trans.* 8, 147-150 (1980).

(37) R. Schoental, "Mycotoxicoses by proxy," *Intern. J. Environ. Studies* 8, 171-175 (1975).

(38) R. Schoental, "Carcinogenic contaminants in foods," in *Dietary Influence on Cancer: Traditional and Modern,* R. Schoental and T.A. Connors (Eds.) (C.R.P. Press Inc., in press).

(39) J. Harwig, P.M. Scott, D.R. Stolz and B.J. Blanchfield, "Toxins of molds from decaying tomato fruit," *Appl. Envir. Microbiol.* 38, 267-274 (1979).

(40) R.F. Vesonder, A. Ciegler, A.H. Hensen, W.K. Rohwedder and D. Weisleder, "Coindentity of the refusal and emetic principle from *Fusarium*-infected corn," *Appl. Environ. Microbiol.* 31, 280-285 (1976).

(41) K.L. Jones and D.W. Smith, "The fetal alcohol syndrome: an epidemiologic perspective," *Teratology* 12, 1-10 (1975).

(42) A.P. Streissguth, S. Landesman-Dwyer, J.C. Martin and D.W. Smith, "Teratogenic effects of alcohol in humans and laboratory animals," *Science* 209, 353-361 (1980).

(43) F.J. Bové, *The Story of Ergot* (Karger, Basel, 1970).

(44) R.C. Shank, "Mycotoxicoses of Man: Dietary and Epidemiological Considerations" in *Mycotoxic Fungi, Mycotoxins, Mycotoxicoses: An Encyclopedic Handbook* 3, T.D. Wylie and L.G. Morehouse (Eds.) (Marcel Dekker, New York, 1978), 1-19.

(45) K. Uraguchi, M. Saito, Y. Noguchi, M. Takahashi, M. Enomoto and T. Tatsuno, "Chronic toxicity and carcinogenicity in mice of the purified mycotoxins, luteoskyrin and cyclochlorotine," *Food Cosmet. Toxicol.* 10, 193-207 (1972).

(46) R. Schoental, "If I had 2500 million pounds to spare on cancer," *Intern. J. Environ. Studies* 15, 65-66 (1980).

(47) J.L. Richard, J.R. Thurston and A.C. Pier, "Effects of mycotoxins on immunity" in *Toxins, Animal, Plant and Microbial,* P. Rosenberg (Ed.), *Toxicon,* Suppl. 1 (Pergamon Press, Oxford, 1978).

(48) Y. Rosenstein, C. Lafarge-Frayssinet, G. Lespinats, F. Loisillier, P. Lafont and C. Frayssinet, "Immunosuppressive acitivity of *Fusarium* toxins. Effects on antibody synthesis and skingrafts of crude extracts, T2-toxin and diacetoxyscirpenol," *Immunology* 36, 111-117 (1979).

13

Role of Zinc, Manganese, Chromium, and Vitamin Deficiencies in Birth Defects

Carl C. Pfeiffer

SUMMARY

The author first considers the aetiology of malnutrition and, then, some aspects of preventative nutrition. A detailed survey follows of nutritional factors and their role in physiology and health, e.g., folic acid, thiamine, pyridoxine, zinc, iron, calcium, magnesium, chromium, copper, fluoride and manganese. The role of suitable nutrition in preparation for parenthood is stressed.

The well-nourished American is a myth. Despite the high level of education and the abundance of available food, many people make poor choices and are badly nourished. Advanced stages of vitamin deficiency diseases still occur in America. Recent evidence has shown that these classic syndromes constitute only a small segment of the total results of malnutrition. Undiagnosed subclinical malnutrition of trace elements and protein may exist and subtly cause much physiological damage to body and brain.

National nutritional surveys have indicated that most people have low levels of one or more essential nutrients relative to the traditionally recommended levels. A study "National Nutrition" at a New Jersey Medical Center was published in "Science" in 1974 and showed that 83% of patients admitted to the hospital have at least one vitamin deficiency and 68% have two or more deficiencies.

AETIOLOGY OF MALNUTRITION

The aetiology of malnutrition may be divided into two categories, primary and secondary. Primary malnutrition results from the faulty or inadequate intake of nutrients by faulty food selection, lack of money, poisoned and contaminated foods, insufficient soil nutrients, or by food shortages. Secondary malnutrition is due to factors interfering with the ingestion, absorption or utilization of essential nutrients, or to stress factors that increase their requirement, destruction or excretion. Primary and secondary malnutrition may exist together, and the effects may be severe and lasting. Adequate nutrition is essential for proper and optimal growth. Kallen asserts that malnutrition during development leads to high infant mortality and smaller physical size.[1] Severe malnutrition may lead to intellectual impairment. However, the relationship between moderate malnutrition and intelligence is still unclear. Winick has illustrated a critical period of the first six months of development during which time cell division takes place and malnutrition may produce irreversible damage.

The late Professor B.S. Platt of The London School of Hygiene and Tropical Medicine found that protein-calorie deficiency during pregnancy in dogs caused neurological dysfunction simulating that of central nervous system damage in human infants. The negative effects of malnutrition on intellectual capacity and on physiological development result in reduction in growth rate, delayed physical maturation, and decreased learning ability. Furthermore, a synergistic interrelationship exists between malnutrition and infectious disease, the two largest world health problems. Infections may be associated with pregnancy and the post-partum state and diabetes. Obviously little help stems from monitoring mother and fetus during the last few days of pregnancy when both have suffered months of malnutrition. Pregnancy is a severe nutritional stress. Ideally, good nutrition should begin many years before pregnancy.

PREVENTATIVE NUTRITION

The statistics show the need for preventative nutrition. A lifetime of better nutrition can contribute significantly to modifying the development of many diseases. According to Dr. Edith Weir, assistant director of USDA's human nutrition research division, diet has played an important role in recent decades in reducing the number of infant and maternal deaths, and deaths from infectious diseases among children.

Emphasis should be placed on a preventive approach to disease rather than on the role of diet in treating health problems after they develop. Most doctors and hospitals are not nutritionally orientated and rarely advise patients about dietary needs. Nutrition receives little attention in the medical school curriculum, and most physicians have not yet recognised that nutrition is an essential part of good medicine. Nutrition is a young science, and our present knowledge about human nutritional needs is limited, especially for conditions such as pregnancy. The gaps in this knowledge are not being filled fast enough. We agree with the view of some doctors that nutrition should properly be a speciality in medicine emphasizing biochemistry and clinical nutrition.[2,3]

For years, representatives of public health groups have promoted that familiar adage, "To enjoy good health, eat a balanced diet." Despite these proclamations, recent nutritional surveys reveal a general ignorance regarding what constitutes a properly balanced diet and, worse still, the fact that even a well-balanced diet can produce borderline or outright deficiencies in one or more of the essential nutrients. Recommended Daily Allowances specify the nutrient allowances necessary for the prevention of severe deficiency diseases, *not* for optimal health. Genetic abnormalities, pregnancy, illness, great occupational stress or drug use often creates a greater need for certain vitamins and trace elements than the sparse quantities specified as RDA's.

Studies by Davis, University of California at Irvine, revealed striking deficits in a diet composed of acceptable staple foods. In a three-month study rats were placed on:

(1) An approximation of the average American diet;

(2) The same diet supplemented with 12 vitamins and 13 trace elements;

(3) Purina Rat Chow; and

(4) Purina Rat Chow diluted with glucose up to 20% of the calories.

Results showed the Rat Chow to be the best diet! The supplemented human diet followed as a close second to the Rat Chow, while rats maintained on the remaining diets trailed behind those of the first two groups in size, physical maturity and general health.

What is wrong with the "well-balanced diet" eaten today? Nutrient deficient soils, chemical fertilizers, time required for shipping and storage, and finally, processing and treatment with chemical additives, deprive plants and animals of vital nutrients as they journey from the farm to the consumer. In 32 states of America the zinc content of soil falls below the adequate level. Plants will continue to grow, despite suboptimal conditions, but suboptimal health will be noted in animals and animals and humans consuming plants raised on deficient soils. Other deficiency syndromes ensue from a lack of other trace elements in the soil.

At the commercial freezing plant, during the freezing process, green vegetables may be scalded with the chelating agent, EDTA, partially removing metals such as zinc, manganese and calcium. Because the surface metals are removed the vegetables will remain a bright green when cooked. Owing to the widespread use of EDTA in food processing in the U.S.A. man may consume as much as 100 mg/day, further affecting the body's intake of trace metals.

Metals are also removed during processing of such foods as peanut butter and oils, and similar losses occur in the refining of cereals and sugar. Each of these foods contains a natural abundance of vitamins, minerals, enzymes, lipids and protein. In processing both become stripped down to devitalized products which are inferior to the whole foods.

Several major deficits result from the removal of vital nutrients from whole wheat and sugar. White flour and sugar supply plenty of calories, but lack the nutrients necessary for the proper utilisation of these calories. Vitamin B_6, vitamin E, chromium, manganese, zinc and magnesium (all removed during processing) play a significant role in the body's use of starches and sugars.[4] Chromium, for example, occurs in the Glucose Tolerance Factor (GTF) needed in sugar metabolism. Chromium levels rise in the blood in response to sugar ingestion, and with each rise, some chromium is lost in the urine. Refined white flour contains only 13% of the chromium found in whole wheat, and refined sugar only a trace of chromium found in sugar cane. Consequently, the body must rely on the chromium content of other foods in order to metabolize carbohydrates. These other foods may not form part of the daily diet.

Processing removes a greater percentage of some minerals than others, thus upsetting the natural balance. For example, whole wheat typically contains cadmium and zinc in a ratio of 1 to 120, but after processing the ratio may be reduced. Cadmium competes with and displaces the vitally important zinc.

FUNCTIONAL HYPOGLYCEMIA

The hypoglycemias have now gained widespread attention. Functional hypoglycemia has been pinpointed as the cause of many everyday emotional problems such as fatigue, depression and irritability, and it is known to contribute in some people to epilepsy, allergies, asthma, ulcers, arthritis, lack of libido in women, impotency in men, suicidal intent, underachievement at school, and hostile or asocial behaviour. Conditions which display a high incidence of hypoglycemia include alcohol or drug addiction, obesity and mental illness.

The hypoglycemic disorders are classified according to whether symptoms occur after eating (reactive hypoglycemia) or when food is withheld (fasting hypoglycemia). Reactive, or functional hypoglycemia, represents about 70% of adult symptomatic hypoglycemia. (In adults fasting hypoglycemia occurs in only a few rare conditions.) The origins of functional hypoglycemia are complex.

Relatively little is known about the mechanisms. We know that in normal people insulin is released from the pancreas in response to raised sugar in the blood after the intake of food. Insulin removes the blood sugar for storage in the liver as glycogen. The polypeptide glucogen, growth hormones, glucocorticoids, and adrenalin are antagonists and raise the blood sugar. We know further that glucogen and/or other factors stimulate the conversion of glycogen from the liver back to glucose and its release into the bloodstream. In this way the proper blood glucose level should be maintained at all times.

Hypoglycemia is probably the result of several malfunctions. Insulin secretion by the normal pancreas stops when the blood glucose concentration falls into the normal hypoglycemia range. In cases of hypoglycemia the delicate balance is not maintained between insulin and the antagonists, which normally regulates the blood sugar. The recently discovered GTF which contains chromium, nicotinic acid and three amino acids, is essential for the proper functioning of insulin. No one is absolutely certain of the cause of the malfunctions resulting in functional hypoglycemia. In some cases it may be due to inborn errors of metabolism. However, it is frequently triggered (in genetically predisposed people) by diet or stress.

The major cause is thought to be the amount of sugar and other refined carbohydrates and stimulants (caffeine, nicotine, etc.) ingested, especially in the United States. The average American consumes between 115 and 150 lb of sugar per capita per year. This is contrasted with the 5 to 10 lb per person per year just 100 to 150 years ago. The body's biochemical processes cannot handle this increased load.

The hypoglycemic response can be triggered by many factors, one of the most important of which is stress. Stress, emotional or physical can result from poor diet, infection, pain, over-exertion, pregnancy, lactation, physical injury, chronic worries, drugs, or alcohol. The stress of pregnancy and childbirth often precipitates hypoglycemia in those women susceptible by constitution or dietary history, resulting in a long-lasting period of postpartum difficulties.

Other causes of functional hypoglycemia are excessive use of tobacco and alcohol, stimulants (coffee, tea, etc.), the birth control pill, or high doses of estrogen, some psycho-tranquillizer drugs and diuretics. These may all disturb the control of the blood sugar level and contribute to hypoglycemia.

The B-Complex vitamins and trace elements are essential for carbohydrate metabolism, and deficiency or poor assimilation of these essential nutrients may contribute. Any disease is made worse by poor nutrition and this certainly includes functional hypoglycemia.

FOLIC ACID (FOLATE)

One of the nutrients found to be essential to normal pregnancy is folic acid. In 1945 Dr. Tom Spies demonstrated that folic acid was effective in the treatment of megaloblastic anemia of pregnancy (and also of tropical sprue). Folic acid is slightly soluble in water, easily oxidised in an acid medium and easily destroyed by sunlight and heat. Much of the folic acid in food can be lost by storage at room temperature and by cooking.

Man must obtain folic acid from dietary sources. It is mostly stored in the liver. Its conversion to folinic acid, the biologically active form, is probably made with aid of ascorbic acid. Folinic acid is a coenzyme for many enzyme systems, much of its activity being interrelated with vitamin B_{12}.

One of the folic acid's most crucial roles is in the synthesis of nucleoproteins, such as DNA and RNA, and thus folate is needed, with vitamin B_{12}, for the production of normal red blood cells in the bone marrow. Deficiency leads to megaloblastic anaemia. Folate also performs an important function in the biosynthesis and transfer of single carbon units such as the methyl group. These processes result in the making of methylated compounds such as choline and other lipotropic substances. The transfer of a methyl group is also essential to one of the components of DNA.

The RDA of folic acid is 0.4 to 0.5 mg/day for adults, 0.8 mg/day for pregnant women and 0.5 mg/day for lactating women. The recommendation during infancy is 0.05 mg to 0.1 mg/day. An individual's requirement will vary with metabolic rate and cellular turnover, and people with hemolytic anaemia or hyperthyroidism need much more.

The average balanced diet contributes 0.15 to 0.2 mg/day, less than half the recommended allowance of 0.5 mg. Many people suffer from borderline folate deficiency. People who eat no green or leafy vegetables are most susceptible. The folic acid level is also related to iron intake. An iron deficiency anaemia will result in lowered plasma folate, and correction with oral iron will establish again the proper balance.[5] When carbohydrate foods constitute too large a proportion of the diet, folate deficiency may develop because these foods contain only traces of folate and iron.

Folate deficiency usually produces irritability, forgetfulness and mental sluggishness. The deficiency may also produce cheilosis, a condition characterised by lesions at the corners of the mouth, which was observed by Rose to be alleviated by folate administration.[6]

The World Health Organisation reports that from one-third to one-half of expectant mothers suffer folic acid deficiency in the last three months of pregnancy.[7] A special need for folic acid exists in pregnancy, as is noted by the approximate doubling of the normal adult RDA. The fetus, by drawing from the mother's folate reserves to meet the needs for rapid growth, often depletes the mother's reserves to the point of megaloblastic anaemia. Many women with histories of abortion and miscarriage have been able to complete successful childbirth subsequent to folic acid supplementation.

Folic acid deficiency in the fetus can produce any of a wide spectrum of congenital anomalies and folate deficiency has also been observed in mentally retarded children.[8,9] Folic acid is thought to be manufactured to some extent by bacteria in the intestinal tract. Prolonged use of antibiotics kills these bacteria and sometimes leads to a lack of both folate and B_{12}. In some women oral contraceptives have produced deficiencies due to decreased absorption. Excessive alcohol consumption accelerates megaloblastic changes; about 90% of alcoholics suffer folic acid deficiencies. Anticonvulsants, such as phenyton or phenobarbital, can produce folate deficiences which lead to a paranoid state.

THIAMINE (VITAMIN B_1)

Thiamine performs several functions, the most important of which is related to carbohydrate metabolism. It is involved to a lesser extent in the metabolism of fats and amino acids. Thiamine aids digestion and elimination by helping to maintain muscle tone in the digestive tract as it does in the heart, is necessary for normal growth and good appetite, and is essential to a healthy nervous system.

Humans need approximately half a milligram of thiamine per thousand calories. Diets high in fats and proteins require somewhat less; however, a minimum allowance of at least 1.0 mg is recommended for all adults. The minimal allowance for pregnant and lactating women is increased by 0.1 and 0.5 mg respectively, beyond the basic requirements.

A potential difficulty in obtaining sufficient thiamine is the vitamin's ready solubility in water and its destruction by heating in a neutral or alkaline reaction. Cooking results in thiamine depletion of most foods. The storage in the body of thiamine is not very great, and tissues are rapidly depleted during a deficiency. Eating sugar, smoking and drinking alcohol further deplete thiamine.

Many Americans do not obtain enough thiamine and may suffer from a mild thiamine deficiency. The 1965 USDA food intake studies indicated that although almost all men got more than the RDA, many adolescent girls and many women over 65 got only about 85% of the RDA.

The symptoms of mild thiamine deficiency are vague and can be attributed to other problems, so that diagnosis is often difficult. Most commonly, the individual experiences fatigue, insomnia, headaches, numbness, neuritis, aching or burning sensations in hands and feet, indigestion, constipation, diarrhoea and loss of appetite, weight and strength. Mental symptoms include apathy, confusion, emotional instability, irritability, depression and fear of impending disaster. Often the mental symptoms are prominent after only a few days of deficiency, and are not accompanied by symptoms or signs of neuritis. Dr. Joseph Brozek of the University of Minnesota has noted significant behavioural decrement in the sensory area with thiamine deprivation.[10] Deterioration of manual speed and co-ordination, complex body-reaction time, toe reaction time, motor speed, eye-hand co-ordination, manual steadiness and body sway were reversed with adequate thiamine supplementation.

RIBOFLAVIN (VITAMIN B$_2$)

Riboflavin is essential to normal growth and tissue maintenance. It goes into the formation of some enzymes and assists in the metabolism of amino acids, fatty acids and carbohydrates, the three energy-generating food constituents.

The RDA of riboflavin is 0.8 to 2.6 mg for adults. During pregnancy and lactation, 1.8 to 2 mg daily are recommended. The individual need will be increased by thyroid disfunction, fevers, stress of injury or surgery, and malabsorption. The yellow riboflavin crystals are resistant to heat, acids and oxidising agents and are only sparingly soluble in water, but they are quickly decomposed by sunlight, ultraviolet rays and alkaline solutions. Much of the *riboflavin in milk is lost* in even one hour of exposure to direct sunlight in a glass container. Three and one-half hours' exposure to the sun's rays will destroy as much as 70%. At maximum, however, 10 to 20% is lost by pasteurisation, evaporation or drying. Opaque containers should increasingly replace glass milk bottles.

Signs of vitamin B$_2$ deficiency are cheilosis and inflammation of the tongue and cornea. Other symptoms are a purple-red tongue; dermatitis around the nose, forehead and ears; eye fatigue, sensitivity to light, blurred vision and bloodshot eyes. The ocular manifestations are often among the earliest warnings of riboflavin deficiency. B$_2$ deficiency can also produce trembling, dizziness insomnia, and mental sluggishness.

One should note that American white flour has had 23 nutrients removed and is then fortified with some of the above vitamins (B$_1$, B$_2$ B$_3$) and iron. (In the U.K., flour is not fortified with Vitamin B$_2$.) A few important give-backs to the flour such as vitamin B$_6$, calcium, magnesium, zinc, and manganese have been proposed. As bureaucracy moves slowly the actual date of further "enrichment" of white flour is unknown. The fortification of flour and cornmeal with nicotinamide has eradicated pellagra, so we predict that the addition of zinc, manganese and vitamin B$_6$ will reduce the incidence of teenage mental disease because pyrroluria will be controlled.

PYRIDOXINE (VITAMIN B$_6$)

Pyridoxine is another one of the water-soluble B-complex vitamins which has a coenzyme involved in an enormous number of reactions. Most of them affect the metabolism of amino acids, the building blocks of proteins. The conversion of tryptophan into NAD is dependent upon pyridoxine and zinc. B$_6$ has importance in red blood cell formation and in central nervous system hormones. Fats, carbohydrates, and all proteins need pyridoxine in order to be utilised in the body. The active form of B$_6$, pyridoxal phosphate, requires zinc in order to get its phosphate group attached. B$_6$ also aids in the absorption of zinc from the intestine. B$_6$ and zinc go together and are more important in the daily diet than salt and pepper. The scientists at the Brain Bio Center were the first to use B$_6$ and zinc/manganese in mental disease. Rimland reported on its use in autistic chilren in 1972.

Along with vitamin B$_3$, Cott (1971) and others have found B$_6$ useful in the treatment of hyperkinetic children. Pfeiffer *et al* (1972, 1974) has shown that kryptopyrrole (formerly known as the mauve factor) binds pyridoxine and zinc. Patients with large quantities of kryptopyrrole will, therefore, exhibit a pyridoxine-deficient state. Patients with krytopyrroluria should be treated with megadoses of pyridoxine combined with zinc and manganese. The usual megadose level is 250 to 2000 mg/day of vitamin B$_6$. The dose can be carefully increased until normal dream recall occurs. B$_6$ should be given in a single morning dose. Doses later in the day can cause insomnia. The mineral factor in dream recall is manganese and Pfeiffer showed that the combination of zinc and manganese is most effective in causing the elimination of excess copper via the urinary pathway.

Pyrroluria is undoubtedly a factor in many birth defects. A notable percentage, probably 10% of men and women, excrete kryptopyrrole when stressed. When kryptopyrrole leaves the body via the urine pyridoxal and zinc are also taken from the body. The zinc-, manganese- and B$_6$-deficient mother will have more nausea and vomiting during the early months of pregnancy. The zinc and manganese is more important in the development of the male fetus so that women who are so deficient will abort male fetus. If the male fetus is carried to term the male baby may be stillborn. If the male baby survives the infant may have birth defects, seizures and end up as a learning disabled child.

The miscarriage of the male fetus results in all-girl families and occasionally all of the girls of the family will have a psychosis which is easily induced by stress. We at The Brain Bio Center have seen many such all-girl families. Later when the young ladies are married and receiving an adequate vitamin B$_6$ with a dietary supplement of zinc and manganese they give birth to normal male children—perhaps the first normal male child in the history of the family.

We have also treated pyrroluria families where the family tree shows predominantly females and the occasional male is mentally retarded. This family curse again responds to adequate zinc/manganese and vitamin B$_6$.

At the Brain Bio Center all "mentally retarded" children and all "learning disabled" children are treated as pyrroluric patients using vitamin B$_6$ and a zinc/manganese supplement.

THE ROLE OF ZINC

With regard to zinc, the American human diet contains only one-tenth that of the 15-25 ppm in animal feed. Soil exhaustion, food processing, careless cooking and the consumption of junk foods all contribute to this low level. Adults should get 15 mg of zinc per day, in pregnancy 20 mg/day, and in lactation 25 mg/day, with 3-5 mg for infants, and 10 mg for chilren aged 1-10 years;[11] but analyses of well-rounded diets served in cafeterias and hospitals show only 8-11 mg/day. Institutional diets are even lower in their total available zinc content.[12]

At present no environmental factor increases our zinc intake. The use of galvanised food processing vessels used to provide some useful zinc contamination, now stainless steel is used. In the case of water pipes, acid water used to take off some of the lining of the galvanized pipes, and provide some zinc, but also some cadmium as the zinc was not pure. Now acid drinking water may provide too much copper from the copper plumbing.

Many factors decrease the effective zinc in food and water in modern society. If the plant, grain, fruit or nut has enough zinc from the soil, then the food will have a normal zinc level. With adequate fertilisation and scientific farming, the zinc should be there for the eating.

While rodents and nocturnal animals have higher levels of zinc in the retina, man in general has higher zinc levels than other animals. If we except the retina and the pineal gland, the highest level of zinc in the brain is in the hippocampus, where histamine is also present. Histamine is stored with zinc.

Several studies have been made of trace metals in the brain. Harrison *et al*, 1968, studied copper, zinc, iron and magnesium distribution.[13] They found copper to be the highest in the caudate nucleus, zinc and magnesium highest in the hippocampus and iron highest in the globus pallidus. Ibata and Otsuka[14] using histochemical techniques, found zinc to be present mainly in the terminal vesicles of the nerve endings of the hippocampal formation of rabbits and rats.

Since zinc occurs with histamine in both basophils and mast cells, one can speculate that the terminal vesicles of the mossy fibres of the hippocampus, may be histaminergic–the nerve impulse may be generated when histamine is released. The hippocampus is an important structure in regard to thoughts, memory and emotions. If the histamine of the histaminergic nerve fibres is stored with zinc, and as histamine appears to be in both the mast cell and the basophil, a functional role in histamine storage could be ascribed to the zinc in the terminal vesicles of the mossy fibres.[15] The use of zinc in the storage of the neurotransmitter, histamine of the hippocampus was suggested in 1971 by Niklowitz.[16] Haug *et al*, in the same year, found that the depletion of zinc in the hippocampus after degeneration of the mossy fibres is compatible with the concept of a neurotransmitter role for zinc.[17] McLardy, 1973, found a decrease in the cells of the hippocampus in both schizophrenics and alcoholics.[18] Any deficiency in mossy fibre cells, or of zinc or histamine in the cells might result in schizophrenic behaviour.

While the original studies on zinc deficiency in males disclosed infantile sex organs, dwarfism and anaemia, we know that many more signs and symptoms of zinc deficiency can be detected by the informed clinical observer. The skin may show striae over the hips, thighs, abdomen, breasts and shoulder girdle.

The B_6 and zinc-deficient teenage girl may not have an established menstrual cycle until age 15 to 17. Painful knee and hip joints may plague the teenager who is zinc deficient. The healing of wounds or burns may be delayed. There may be loss of taste (hypogeusia) and severe depression.

The nauseated pregnant woman is also usually deficient in both vitamin B_6 and zinc. Both are needed for growing tissues of any kind and the fetus in the uterus makes extraordinary demands on the mother's supply. Vitamin B_6 has been used for nausea and vomiting of pregnancy with uneven success. We have had many pregnant patients who had difficulty with previous pregnancies go through a pregnancy on a zinc and B_6 regime with no difficulties.

Several workers, notably Dr. Lucille Hurley, University of California, have shown that zinc deficiency in pregnant rats will result in many stillborn pups, and that those born may have one of a number of birth defects.[19] Caldwell *et al* have shown that the rats born to mildly zinc- or manganese-deficient mothers are mentally retarded and do not learn as well as rats born to zinc-supplemented mothers.[20],[21] Colleagues visiting Iran and Egypt are told that 30% of the young children are slow learners. It may not be a concidence that these areas of the world which have been farmed for centuries no longer have much available zinc in the soil.[22]

For more than 50 years New Zealand agriculturalists have sought effective means of preventing and treating a fatal disease which afflicts farm animals in their country during the autumn. The disease is caused by a fungus toxin found in certain grasses and produces liver damage and severe facial eczema.

Recent studies, based on the observations of Gladys Reid,[23] indicate that zinc sulphate is an effective prophylactic. Reid has for long been concerned over the numbers of New Zealand breeding stock that develop difficulties late in pregnancy. Extreme muscular weakness, a teetering walk, failure to eat enough and gain weight, eczema on the face and at the base of the tail, failure to lift the tail with subsequent soiling and lethargy precalving are symptoms of the disorder, termed "sulky cow syndrome." If the animal does not collapse in the last week of pregnancy she will produce a dead or weak calf after a prolonged and stressful labour. Reid has found that animals who suffer this condition can be revived by coaxing them to eat hay soaked in molasses and a special proprietary stock meal, both extremely high in zinc. Reid was familiar with the studies of Jean Apgar of the U.S.A. Agricultural Research Service which showed that zinc-deficient laboratory animals suffer considerable lethargy in advanced pregnancy and have a long and difficult labour.[24]

Reid began administering zinc sulphate to her "sulky" cows. Given one teaspoonful (about 5 gm) of zinc sulphate even the most seriously ill animals were on their feet in hours, their appetites returned in several days, and they gave birth to healthy calves.

Zinc is stored in the liver and Reid observed that the collapse of the cow with the toxin-induced liver damage occurred at the same time and in the same manner as the collapse of the zinc-deficient animal at the birth of young. Reid has also found zinc supplementation beneficial for improving the general health and disposition of young animals. Reid's observations interested Towers *et al* of the Ruarura Agricultural Research Center, N.Z. In studies these scientists found that rats fed diets deficient in zinc became severely ill and died shortly after administration of the fungus toxin, while rats fed diets supplemented with zinc escaped serious liver damage when the fungus toxin was administered, and survived. In field trials using sheep and milking cows large doses of oral zinc sulphate reduced liver damage following administration of the fungus toxin. The New Zealand workers conclude that oral zinc sulphate in large doses will protect farm animals against the fungus toxin.

In another study, B.F. Rickard divided 50 yearling calves affected with facial eczema into two groups. Twenty-five calves were treated with oral zinc sulphate while the remaining calves served as controls.[25] Within ten days the treated group showed considerable improvement. The animals' skin lesions were healing well, they gained weight and their coats began to shine. Animals in the control group failed to improve and many died.

IRON DEFICIENCY

Iron is essential to human body chemistry since it combines with protein to make haemoglobin. The body makes efficient use of iron stores by recycling, but when blood is lost through menstruation or haemorrhage, iron is also lost, and must be replaced by adequate dietary intake. Iron overload is most likely to occur in older men, as the excess iron accumulates gradually over the years. Iron deficiency is more likely to occur in women than in men and in teenagers whose rapid growth may require additional iron. In pregnancy, and cases of overt blood loss, the risk of deficiency is enough to merit supplements. Research has revealed that iron absorption in the human body is complex, but acids such as malic and ascorbic do promote absorption.[26,27] For this reason iron deficiency anaemia is variably responsive to iron supplementation depending on what is eaten with the iron.

In a study of 300 pregnant women, dosages of 100 to 200 mg of ferrous sulphate resulted in the same rise in haemoglobin levels. Other nutritional factors affect iron absorption. Vitamin C supplements increase iron absorption significantly, and eggs and orange juice in the mornings are recognised as a nutritionally advantageous combination. Vitamin C in the orange juice reduces the iron of egg yolk, facilitating its absorption. An unbalanced vegetarian diet, or excess consumption of phosphate results in less iron being absorbed.[28] The toxic metals lead and cadmium reduce iron absorption.[29]

CALCIUM BALANCE

Some 99% of the calcium in the body is found in the bones. The other 1% is just as vital because it is involved in controlling blood clotting mechanisms, the excitability of nerves and muscles, the function of the parathyroid hormone and the action of vitamin D.

Calcium occurs in the blood, the fluid surrounding cells, cell membranes and intracellular organelles. Unfortunately, according to a survey released in 1968 by the USDA, over 30% of the population of the U.S.A. is calcium deficient. (This statement contradicts the conventional medical view that calcium deficiency is in practice prevented from occurring by the homeostatic mechanisms which are supposed to regulate calcium metabolism.) The National Academy of Sciences states that men, women and children (aged one to ten) need 800 mg of calcium daily. Infants need only 360 to 540 mg, while growing boys and girls, and pregnant and lactating women need 1200 mg daily. Lukens considers that 1000 mg of calcium daily in older people may completely prevent osteoporosis.[30]

Regardless of age, whether a person is ingesting adequate calcium or not, the body will lose this mineral every day. Approximately 100 to 200 mg of calcium is filtered from the blood and excreted in the urine. An additional 125 to 180 mg is excreted in the digestive juices, remains unabsorbed and passes out of the body in the faeces. Also a small amount is lost in sweat.

Calcium is essential, but its interaction with other vitamins and minerals must not be overlooked. A lack of magnesium can cause calcium deposits in muscles, heart and kidney which may result in kidney stones. Enough B_6 to produce recall of dreams will allow enough pyridoxic acid to form to prevent kidney stones of the calcium oxalate type. Many urologists put their stone-forming patients on some vitamin B_6 but success depends on a dose adequate to ensure that some goes over into the urine as pyridoxic acid.

Milk is ordinarily the best source of a balanced solution of calcium, magnesium and phosphorus. Two glasses of milk per day should be drunk by every growing individual and every pregnant woman. One eight-ounce glass per day should be drunk by every adult, and if this rule is followed the adult will not lose the ability to use lactose or milk sugar. Some 20% of white adults and 80% of black adults may have impaired ability to digest lactose, mainly because they stopped using milk in early childhood.

Dolomitic calcium and magnesium can be used by the adult who is sensitive to milk. Since the magnesium makes the calcium soluble, the danger of kidney stones which occur with calcium alone is eliminated.

Calcium deficiency is marked by increased nervousness and bone weakness. Osteomalacia has been associated with use of anticonvulsants which are antifolate and also accelerate the breakdown of vitamin D. A vitamin D deficiency results in impaired calcium absorption. For example, calcium-deficient mothers give birth to children with reduced bone density.[31] A deficiency in calcium also plays an important role in cardiac arrythmias. Calcium is functionally important for many cardiac cells and is primarily responsible for generation of the electrical potential in the conducting system.

Calcium supplements such as bone meal, dolomite, calcium lactate or milk are good and healthy ways to promote sleep, though some samples of bone meal have been found to contain potentially dangerous levels of the toxic element lead, the metabolic handling of which mimics that of calcium.[32]

MAGNESIUM BALANCE

The National Academy of Sciences has set the RDA for magnesium at 350 mg for men, 300 mg for women, and 450 mg during pregnancy and lactation.

Magnesium is steadily declining in the American diet with the refining and processing of food. Characteristics of deficiency are muscle tremors, convulsions, depression, poor memory, delirium and heart irregularities. Rats fed a *magnesium-deficient diet* give birth to smaller rats with *more congenital malformations,* and they develop calcium deposits and other abnormalities within the heart cells.

Magnesium deficiency in man is difficult to diagnose because of the ambiguity of the physiological symptoms–humans maintain normal blood, serum and CSF magnesium levels even on a magnesium-deficient diet. As much as half the magnesium stored in bones may be released before a decrease in blood serum will occur. Magnesium is needed for mobilisation of calcium from bone. Most calcium and magnesium stores are in the skeletal system. A suggested test for deficiency is the intravenous injection of excess magnesium; a normal person excretes 90% of this, while a deficient person excretes less and absorbs more.

Magnesium deficiencies are often accompanied by hypocalcaemia and hypokalaemia (low potassium). There are many similarities between potassium and magnesium metabolism, although magnesium is much harder to displace from a cell than potassium. The concentration of potassium in cells is reduced by magnesium deficiency and does not return to normal until this has been corrected. Many dietary causes of magnesium deficiency are also causes of potassium deficiencies. Calcium supplements without adequate magnesium cannot prevent hypocalcaemia.

Magnesium salts, the bicarbonate, carbonate, oxide, chloride and sulphate, all have been successful in treating deficiencies. (A calcium source is needed with a prolonged dose of any of these salts.) Magnesium sulphate therapy has been particularly successful in treating convulsions of newborn babies.[33] The best dietary supplement is probably dolomite with pure bone meal, which provides adequate magnesium, calcium, phosphorus and other trace elements. Bone meal should not be used as the exclusive source of calcium, for such use can rarely cause lead poisoning.

People living in regions with hard drinking water (plenty of magnesium and calcium carbonates) have a reduced risk of magnesium deficiency. These hard water areas also have a lessened incidence of heart disease and atherosclerosis.[34]

THE NEED FOR ORGANIC CHROMIUM

In Western countries the body content of chromium decreases with age, while in Eastern countries where natural foods are eaten the chromium content is maintained.[35]

Many women in Western countries are so deficient in chromium that the white blood cell chromium level may decrease by 50% with each pregnancy, resulting first in complete alcohol intolerance and later in glucose intolerance (adult-type diabetes). The best two sources of chromium are brewer's yeast and sugar beet molasses. Beet molasses is seldom marketed and that leaves brewer's yeast as the best available source.

Humans, like rats, need the Glucose Tolerance Factor (GTF). GTF[36] is an organic chromium compound whose exact chemical structure is now being determined. Trivalent chromium is known to be the centre of the molecule which also contains two niacin molecules and three amino acids, glutamic acid, glycine and cysteine.

GTF is then a trivalent chromium in an organic chemical complex which cannot be easily synthesized in the body, but may be synthesized by the normal bacteria of the intestine when enough chromium is contained in the diet. People in Western nations are depleted of their GTF and need a good dietary source.

Simple measurements of the chromium content of food can be misleading because chromium occurs in several forms with the range of oral absorption between 1 and 10%. Inorganic chromium is only 1% absorbable. Eggs have a high chromium concentration but little of their chromium content is in the organic form biologically available as GTF. Chromium containing foods with biologically active chromium are brewer's yeast, black pepper, liver, beef, wholewheat bread, beets, beet sugar molasses, mushrooms, and beer. Among these, far and away the highest in chromium content is brewer's yeast. For the patient suspected of impaired glucose tolerance, brewer's yeast tablets are an indispensable supplement to the diet.

Chromium has been found to be essential to both the growth and longevity of laboratory animals. Studies done on mice and rats showed that male mice and rats receiving 2 or 5 ppm chromium in their drinking water grew significantly better than their controls. The median age of the male mice and rats was 99 and 91 days longer, respectively than the control animals. No such effect was detected for females. Another site of chromium action is the eye. Rats ingesting low chromium and protein diets developed an opaque cornea and congestion of the iridial vessels.

In man, chromium deficiency may be a factor in arteriosclerosis and hypertension. In addition to disturbing glucose and lipid (cholesterol) metabolism it affects (inhibits) protein synthesis. The amino acids most affected by chromium deficiency are α-aminoisobutyric acid, serine, and methionine.[37] While it is difficult to analyse chromium nutrition in humans, hair analysis has provided a useful comparison of chromium nutritional status since changes in chromium concentration seem to parallel those in other tissues.[38] Evaluation of urine excretion can also indicate deficiencies. Chromium-deficient patients do not have the customary increase in urinary chromium excretion following oral glucose.

Although inorganic tervalent chromium compounds (*e.g.*, $CrCl_3$) are poorly absorbed (1 to 3%) they are very effective in treating kwashiorkor children and marasmic (progressive emaciation) infants. In normal patients there is usually a three-week delay before the inorganic chromium takes effect, although in one case the effect of $CrCl_3$ was immediate. Note that hexavalent chromium compounds (*e.g.*, chromates) are highly toxic and must not be used in therapy.

Long-term studies on GTF have revealed a number of its properties and actions. For example, GTF is non-toxic, it most resembles a hormone, and it is released into the blood in response to insulin and is then transported to the periphery of the insulin target tissue where it promotes better sugar utilisation.[39]

The availability of circulatory chromium appears to decrease during any acute infection. The body's use of chromium to inhibit antibody responses could explain the altered glucose tolerance curve characteristic of infections.[40]

COPPER AS A TRACE ELEMENT

Copper is essential in small amounts in the biosynthesis of haemoglobin, although haemoglobin itself contains no copper. This discovery was made by E.B. Hart of the University of Wisconsin in 1928, but work on the intimate metabolism of copper is proceeding slowly. Traces of copper can be found in medicinal iron preparations and many foods, so adult man seldom suffers from copper deficiency, especially now that copper water pipes have become so common.

At the Brain Bio Center we have determined serum copper in more than 12,000 patients and have not found a single case of copper deficiency. Only premature infants and patients on parenteral (intravenous) feedings have shown such deficiency. The body of an adult typically contains about 125 mg of copper: the liver, via the bile is the main route of excretion of excess copper. The liver has the highest copper content, the brain is second, and other organs and tissues contain much less. Fetal liver at term contains approximately seven times the concentration of copper as is found normally in adult liver. 5 to 15 years are needed to bring the level of copper down to adult level. Since copper is a stimulant to the brain, this excess copper may be a factor in hyperactivity in children, a condition which ameliorates with age and slow elimination of the copper burden. This high level of copper in the young is also evident in sheep and cows. Lamb's liver and calf's liver are much higher in copper than are the livers from full-grown animals.

Levels of copper and particularly the copper-containing enzyme ceruloplasmin in the blood are elevated by estrogens; therefore the levels of copper and ceruloplasmin rise progressively during pregnancy. Serum copper is approximately 115 mg/dl at conception, and reaches a mean of 260 mg/dl at term. After delivery, a period of two to three months is required before the original serum copper level is reached. In the last trimester of pregnancy, zinc accumulates in the placenta. In the animal kingdom, where the placenta is consumed after birth, it is to be presumed the copper/zinc ratio is restored sooner.[41]

This high post-partum copper level may be a factor in causing post-partum depression and psychosis; more data are needed. One must also discover the differences in copper level when a schizophrenic patient carries a male or female child. We know the incidence of post-partum psychosis is much greater after the birth of a male child. If the estrogen level alone were the cause, one would expect the reverse.

According to Ylostalo and Ylikorkala, the exaggerated rise in serum copper may be a factor in toxaemia of pregnancy (pre-eclampsia level 287 mg/dl as against 258 mg/dl for normals)[42] and in hepatosis (inflamation and enlargement of the liver) of pregnancy (serum copper 342 mg/dl). Pfeiffer and Iliev have found that the oral contraceptive, with its potent estrogen, raises copper in schizophrenics to a level higher than that of the ninth month of pregnancy. This rise produces activation of their psychoses, which may last for several weeks after stopping the pill. The remission of the psychoses corresponds to the slow decline of accumulated copper in the blood and tissues.

In sub-acute poisoning of rats with copper, Lal *et al*, have found great increase in liver copper and some deaths. The activity of a zinc-containing enzyme, lactic acid dehydrogenase, was decreased, as were the brain amine oxidases. (Editor's note: This is surprising since many amine oxidases are cuproenzymes.) Brain copper increased 36% in a six-week period, and the turnover of serotonin was apparently reduced. The adrenal glands markedly increased in weight—an index of stress.[43] The changes in copper and iron storage which occur during pregnancy, suckling, and infancy were reviewed by Linder and Munro in 1973. We know that during the suckling period breast milk contains little copper and iron; the amount of copper and iron stored in the infant's liver should therefore decrease in the first six months of life. At this time the liver produces the normal copper protein, ceruloplasmin, which stores copper in the blood serum and prevents excess absorption. Similarly ferritin, the iron-containing protein, is made. Any abnormality which results in inadequate ceruloplasmin or ferritin could allow excess copper or iron to be absorbed, which would affect the brain; both of these metals are stimulants to the brain and might produce hyperactivity, with faulty mental development into adulthood. Nothing in the fetal development process protects against excess copper or iron.

An alternative hypothesis is that aluminum, or heavy metals such as lead, silver, or mercury could interfere with the synthesis of ceruloplasmin or ferritin.

HEART DISEASE AND COPPER

Cases of myocardial infarction in people under 40 are increasing in the United States. The recent studies of Dr. Oscar Roth of the Yale University School of Medicine reveal that the rate is 27 times higher in men than in women, but that women on oral contraceptive medication may have a much greater risk. He has observed five tragic cases of myocardial infarction in women on the pill. Serum copper is high with the use of the birth control pill, and the copper level of the heart is higher than normal in those dying from heart attacks.[44] Copper is also high in patients with high blood pressure and in those who smoke. We therefore can postulate that the smoking woman, on oral contraceptives, whose drinking water is soft acid water which has coursed through copper plumbing, and who is at the same time under stress may have the greatest susceptibility to heart attacks and strokes.

Most of the hypertensive patients we see at the Brain Bio Center have low zinc and high serum copper. As zinc and vitamin C are given, both the lead and copper levels decrease. We cannot measure cadmium, but that is also possibly lowered by zinc and vitamin C therapy. The decrease in copper and lead is accompanied by a *significant decrease in the elevated pressure*, usually to the normal level. Negroes tend to have higher copper and lead levels than whites, and their hypertension is harder to treat. The black or skin tan pigment melanin has a great affinity for copper, a fact which might contribute to the high copper and blood pressure in many blacks.

FLUORIDE IN WATER

The value of fluoride in human nutrition is controversial and the literature on it is marked by contradiction. For every positive assertion as to its value there is a corresponding denial; hence the health profession is divided into those who claim fluoridation of the water supply is poison and those who call it a panacea. The debate focuses on the role of fluoride in bone development and maintenance, and in dental health. Other topics that are disputed, though less studied, are the role of fluoride in cancer, heart disease, congenital malformations, and fluoride intoxication. Many studies have examined the incidence of dental caries in populations with non-fluoridated water supplies versus fluoridated water, or with high fluoride diets versus low fluoride diets. These studies have confirmed a lower rate of caries formation and the possibility of long-lasting benefit. However, most of these studies have ignored the fact that the high fluorine diet results in initial delay wherein fluoride affects the tooth germ, causing a delay in dentition. Schatz has shown that dental caries develop at the same rate in the permanent teeth of fluoridated and non-fluoridated children.[45] A maximum of 10% reduction in caries occurs in children whose teeth developed while they were drinking fluoridated water. While the protective effect of fluoride is hotly debated, it seems to be agreed that once the permanent teeth have fully formed and emerged, high fluoride intake no longer has any effect.

A comparison of cancer rates in the ten largest U.S. cities fluoridated before 1966 with rates of the ten largest cities during the pre-fluoride period, 1944 to 1950, and not fluoridated as from 1969, demonstrated a significant increase in the incidence of cancer and cancer death in fluoridated cities.

A similar study, however, detected no difference in cancer rates between fluoridated and non-fluoridated U.S. counties. The problems inherent in both studies are manifold.[46,47] Claims as to the role of fluoride in heart and vascular conditions have also been contradictory. Similar population studies, as above, have shown both increases and no association between water fluoridation and these conditions.

Another debate centers upon the possible correlation between congenital malformations and a fluoridated water supply. Schatz has reported that fluoridation of the water supply in Chilean cities increased infant mortality and congenital malformations by as much as 288%. On the other hand, a study in the U.S.A. of a comparison of metropolitan Atlanta to several other metropolitan areas showed no association of congenital malformations with fluoridated areas. The differences in findings may relate to the basic nutrition in each population. The Chileans of Curico are relatively malnourished, and hence would be more susceptible to the dangers of fluoride.

MANGANESE NUTRITION

Manganese is another of the essential trace metals, a necessary dietary constituent obtained from nuts, seeds and whole grain cereals. It is necessary for bone growth and development, reproduction, lipid metabolism and the moderation of nervous irritability. Manganese is also important in the building and breakdown cycles of protein and nucleic acids (the chief carriers of genetic information). As an activator of such enzymes as arginase (required for the formation of urea) and some peptidases (which cause the hydrolysis of proteins in the intestine) manganese may also contribute to a mother's love and instinctive protection of her child. Through certain enzymes, manganese affects the glandular secretions underlying maternal instinct. Thus Orent and McCollum reported in 1931 that normal maternal instincts such as nest-building, retrieval, hovering, and nursing were impaired in manganese-deficient mother rats.[20] Manganese is important in the formation of thyroxin, the iodine-containing hormone of the thyroid gland.

Every day a healthy person excretes approximately 4 mg of manganese; this amount is then needed in the diet for the replacement of the lost manganese. Adequate intake is required for the lipid and glucose metabolism and oxidative phosphorylation (and other intrinsic biochemical processes). On normal lipid metabolism, manganese has a beneficial effect, particularly in cases of atherosclerosis.

Analysis of hair samples has indicated that manganese deficiency may be common. Manganese deficiency is suspected in diabetes. Kosenko in 1964 implicated manganese deficiency after an examination of 122 diabetics from 15 to 21 years of age. Kosenko found that the manganese content of whole ashed blood was approximately half that of normal control subjects. In 1968 Everson and Scrader reported that manganese deficiency can impair glucose metabolism so as to lower glucose tolerance. The deficiency may produce abnormalities in the pancreatic secretion of insulin. A diabetic condition may result.

The enzymes that manganese activates are also necessary for the utilisation of vitamin C, choline, thiamin, and biotin. Without the ability to use choline or decanol (2-dimethylaminoethanol) properly, the body underproduces acetylcholine, a neurotransmitter in the brain. In a body deficient in acetylcholine and properly utilized B vitamins, various conditions may result, among them myasthenia gravis. This condition may respond to manganese if doses are given at each meal, in addition to a high protein diet, vitamin E and all the B vitamins. All these nutrients aid the transmission of impulses between nerve and muscle.

Manganese metabolism is similar to that of iron. Manganese is absorbed slowly in the small intestine, and the unneeded portion is excreted. The absorbed portion is transported through the blood by the protein transmanganin; the manganese quickly leaves the bloodstream and is stored mainly in the kidney. Some is excreted in the urine, most into the bile.

Manganese is removed from the soil by soil erosion, leaching, and soil exhaustion, which deplete the amount available to vegetables. This depletion of soil may be unsuspected since the foliage of plants can be lush without manganese. This is typified by the growth of lettuce. If lime is applied to solid clay, leafy vegetables grown in the more alkaline soil will contain much less manganese for calcium is a manganese antagonist. This finding emphasises the very real need for scientific farming, wherein the fertilizer will contain all the trace elements in which the soil is deficient. The germ or bran of the grain contains most manganese, but this is lost in the milling process. White flour contains 9%

of the manganese found in whole wheat. Also, note the drastic losses of manganese from corn; corn germ 10 ppm, corn 1 ppm, corn flakes 0.04 ppm.[48]

Except for the organ meats (such as liver), protein is not a good source of manganese. Fish is low, except for shellfish such as clams or snails. The daily requirement for man is about 4 mg.

The absorptions of iron and manganese are inversely related. High iron in the diet inhibits manganese absorption, and, conversely, high manganese intake inhibits iron absorption in several animal species including man. This relationship also holds for calcium and zinc. Calcium affects absorption and retention of manganese.

Manganese deficiency affects both man and animals. For example, it reduces blood clotting response to extra vitamin K in chickens. Manganese catalyzes the aggregation of human platelets *in vitro*. The manganese iron has an essential role in blood clotting and functions somewhere in the chain prior to direct vitamin K action.[49]

Manganese stimulates adenylate cyclase activity in brain and other tissues of the body as demonstrated in numerous experiments. In one study the striate cortex of rats was tested as a focus of manganese-catalyzed enzyme activity in this region of the brain. This study has great importance because cyclic-AMP plays a regulatory role in the action of several brain neurotransmitters. Thus it was concluded that manganese has an important role in brain function.[50,51] Manganese-deficient female rats and chickens have defective ovulation and their offspring increased mortality. Deficient male rats and rabbits have a loss of libido, lack of semen, and seminal tubule degeneration. The site of manganese action in the reproductive system is as yet unknown. Cotzias in 1958 described manganese-deficient chicks with decreased bone growth, skeletal abnormalities and changes in the CNS. In a number of different species of experimental animals over a wide range of studies, Hill 1950, Everson 1959, Hurley 1958, O'Dell 1961 and Apgar 1968 have found ataxia, poor balance, skeletal malformations, lack of co-ordination, head retraction, loss of righting reflexes, stillbirth and pre-weaning mortality.

CONCLUSION

To conclude, no shortage of any one nutrient is wholly without effect in the experimental animal and in man. Owing to the interdependency and interaction of nutrients one with another, many of these effects may be far-reaching and in some cases irreversible. Where this applies in the adult, the changes may be reflected in the germ cell or in the ovum. Gross deficiencies may result in infertility, and less drastic alterations may result in various forms of foetal damage. The role of nutrition in preparation for parenthood should assume a much greater importance than has applied hithertofore.

This paper is reprinted from the *Intern. J. Environ. Studies* (vol. 17, No. 1, 43-56, May 1981) by kind permission of the publishers Gordon and Breach Ltd., 42 William IV Street, London WC 2 (U.K.). The editor is grateful to the publishers, Gordon and Breach Ltd., for their kind permission to publish this important paper. (Editor)

REFERENCES

(1) D.J. Kallen, "Nutrition and society," *J. Amer. Med. Assoc.* 215, No. 1, 94 (1971).

(2) Editorial "American nutrition: ignorance in abundance," *Medical World News* 6, (1973).

(3) T. Brewer, "Total blackout on role of malnutrition," *Medicine* (1973).

(4) H.A. Schroeder, "Losses of vitamins and trace minerals resulting from processing and preservation of food," *Amer. J. Clin. Nutrition* 24, 562-567 (1971).

(5) A. Omar, N. Finlayson, D. Shearman, R. Samson and R. Girdwood, "Plasma and erythrocyte folate in iron deficiency and folate deficiency," *Blood* 35, No. 6, 821 (1970).

(6) J. Rose, "Folic acid deficiency as a cause of angular cheilosis," *Lancet* 2, 453 (1971).

(7) M. Kruger, "Folic acid requirements during pregnancy," *J. Amer. Med. Assoc.* 218, No. 5, 747 (1971).

(8) R.H. Williams, "Prenatal nutrition," *The Physican's Handbook of Nutritional Science, American Lecture Sorion,* 33 34 (1975).

(9) "Teratogenic effects of some purine analogues in fetal rats," *Archives of Pathology* 86, 396-402 (1968).

(10) J. Brozek, "Societal studies on nutrition and higher nervous system activity," *Annals of the New York Academy of Science* 93, 687 (1962).

(11) *Recommended Dietary Allowances,* 8th edition (Nat. Acad. Sci., Washington, DC, U.S.A., 1974).

(12) E.D. Brown, M.A. McGuckin, M. Wilson and J.C. Smith, Jn., "Zinc in selected hospital diets," *J. Amer. Dietet. Assoc.* 69, 6 (1976).

(13) W.W. Harrison, M.G. Netsky and M.D. Brown, "Trace elements in human brain: copper, zinc, iron and magnesium," *Clinica Chimica Acta* 21, 50-60 (1968).

(14) Y. Ibata and N. Otsuka, "Electron microscopic demonstration of zinc in hippocampus formation using Timm's sulfide-silver technique," *J. Compar. Neurology* 142, 23-31 (1971).

(15) E. Fjerdingstad, G. Danscher and E.J. Fjerdingstad, "Zinc content in hippocampus and whole brain of normal rats," *Brain Research* 79, 338-347 (1974).

(16) W.J. Niklowitz, "Interference of Pb and Mg with essential brain tissue Cu, Fe and Zn as a main determinant in experimental metal encephalopathy," presented at *The Trace Elements and Brain Function Symposium* Princeton, NJ (1973).

(17) F.M. Haug, "Timm's sulphide-silver reaction for zinc during experimental anterograde degeneration of hippocampal mossy fibres," *J. Compar. Neurology* 142, 23-31 (1971).

(18) T. McLardy, "Hippocampal zinc and structural deficit in brain from schizophrenics and chronic alcoholics," presented at *The Trace Elements and Brain Function Symposium,* Princeton, NJ (1973).

(19) L.S. Hurley, "The consequences of fetal impoverishment," *Nutrition Today* 3, 2 (1968).

(20) D. Oberleas, D.F. Caldwell and A.S. Prasad, "Trace elements and behaviour," *Intern. Rev. Neurobiol. Supplement* 1, 83-102 (1972).

(21) D.F. Caldwell, D. Oberleas and A.S. Prasad, "Reproductive performance of chronic mildly zinc deficient rats," *Nutrition Reports Intern.* 7, No. 5, 309-319 (1973).

(22) A.S. Prasad, *Zinc Metabolism* (Chas. C. Thomas, Springfield, Il, 1966).

(23) Mrs. Reid (personal communications).

(24) J. Apgar, "Effect of zinc repletion late in gestation on parturition in the zinc deficient rat," *J. Nutrit.* 103 (1973).

(25) B.F. Rickard, "Facial eczema: zinc responsiveness in dairy cattle," *New Zealand Veterin. J.* 23, 41-42 (1975).

(26) G. Greve *et al*, "Effects of meals and ascorbic acid in the absorption of therapeutic dose of iron as ferrous and ferric salts," *Current Therapeutic Research* 17, 382-397 (1975).

(27) M. Layrisse, "Dietary iron absorption," *Nutrition* 1, 141-148 (1975).

(28) J.E. Sjosedt *et al*, "Oral iron prophylaxis during pregnancy, a comparative study on different dosage regimes," *Acta Obstetrica et Gynecologica Scandinavica* 60, 3-9 (1977).

(29) Editoral "Physical acceptability and bioavailability of iron fortified food, *Nutrition Revs.* 34, 298-300 (1976).

(30) J.N. Lukens, "Iron deficiency and infection," *Amer. J. Diseases of Children* 129, 160-162 (1975).

(31) K.A.V.R. Krishnamachari and L. Irengar, "Effect of maternal malnutrition on the bone density of the neonates," *Amer. J. Clin. Nutrit.* 28, 482-486 (1975).

(32) W.H. Crosby, "Lead contaminated health food: association with lead poisoning and leukaemia," *J. Amer. Med. Assoc.* 237, 2627-2629 (1977).

(33) T.L. Turner *et al*, "Magnesium therapy in neonatal tetany," *The Lancet* 283-294 (1977).

(34) M.S. Seelig, "Electrographic patterns of magnesium depletion appearing in alcoholic heart disease," *Annals of the New York Academy of Sciences* 162, No. 2, 906-917 (1969).

(35) K.M. Hambidge, "Chromium nutrition in man," *Amer. J. Clin. Nutrit.* 27, 505 (1974).

(36) W. Mertz, "Chromium occurrence and function in biological systems," *Phys. Rev.* 49, (1969).

(37) W. Mertz, "Effects and metabolism of glucose tolerance factor," *Nutrition Revs.* 33, No. 5, 129-135 (1975).

(38) J.R. Mahalko and M. Bennion, "The effect of parity and time between pregnancies on maternal hair chromium concentration," *Amer. J. Clin. Nutrit.* 29, 1069-1072 (1976).

(39) E.J. Underwood, *Trace Elements in Human and Animal Nutrition* (New York Academic Press, pp. 258-269, 1977).

(40) R.S. Pecarek *et al*, "Relationship between serum chromium concentrations and glucose utilization in normal infected subjects," *Diabetes* 24, No. 4, 350-353 (1975).

(41) B. Vallee, chapter "Zinc," *Mineral Metabolism* edited by Comar and Bronner (. . . . . 1971).

(42) P. Ylostalo and O. Ylikorkala, "Hepatosis of pregnancy, a clinical study of 107 patients," *Annales Chirugiae et Gynaecologiae Fenniae* 64, 128-134 (1975).

(43) S. Lal, R. Papeschi, R.J.S. Duncan and T.L. Sourkes, "Effects of copper loading on various tissue enzymes and brain mono-amines in the rat," *Toxicology and Applied Pharmacology* 28, 395-405 (1974); M. Liner and H.N. Munro, *Enzyme* 15, 111-113 (1973).

(44) O. Roth, "Myocardial infarct rate rises among young in U.S.," *Intern. Med. News* (1974).

(45) A. Schatz, "Increased death rates in Chile associated with artificial fluoridation of drinking water with implications for other countries," *J. Arts. Sciences and Humanities* 2, No. 1, 11-16 (1976).

(46) R.N. Hoover *et al*, "Fluoridated drinking water and the occurrence of cancer," *J. Cancer* 57, No. 4, 757-768 (1976).

(47) M.L. Bierenbaum, "Effect of fluoridated water on serum lipids, ions and cardiovascular disease: mortality rates," *J. Med. Soc. N.J.* 71, No. 9, 663-666 (1974).

(48) G.J. Everson and R.E. Schrader, "Abnormal glucose tolerance in manganese deficient guinea pigs," *J. Nutrit.* 94, 89 (1968).

(49) P.M. Evans and B.M. Jones, "Manganese induced aggregation of human platelets," *Cytobios* 13, 37-44 (1975).

(50) J. Smeyers-velbeke *et al*, "Distribution of manganese in human brain tissue," *Clinica Chimerica Acta* 68, 343-347 (1976).

(51) C.C. Pfeiffer and B. Aston, *Social Rehabilitation of the Schizophrenic by Specific Nutrients* (Brain Bio Center, Princeton, NJ, 1980).

-14-

Trace Substances in Foods and Their Effect on Health

George V. James

SUMMARY

Trace elements in nutrition are first mentioned together with some illustrations of results of deficiencies. This has been done with particular reference to metallic elements and is followed by referring to the effects of more complex substances such as phytic acid. The presence of cyanogenetic glucosids in various vegetables especially certain pulses and brassica as well as avoidance of ill effects by careful cooking are discussed, while finally the more recent poisoning cases due to consumption of Scombroid fish are mentioned with suggestions as to the causes of these outbreaks.

INTRODUCTION

This paper was given at the conference on "Nutrition and Killer Diseases" (London, 1979). Nutrition was defined as the means of sustaining life as well as to replace tissue loss, to promote growth and to provide energy. In brief, it may be said to be the study of consumed food values.

Health is a state of complete physical, mental and social well-being and not merely the absence of disease or infirmity. The presence or absence of many elements, or substances, in our diets may lead to a person being below "par" or may even result in the development of a disease.

EFFECTS OF CERTAIN ELEMENTAL SUBSTANCES

The following criteria are necessary and sufficient to establish whether an element is essential for the nutrition and well-being of an organism.

    (a) The organism may neither grow nor complete its life cycle without the element.

(b) The particular element cannot be replaced by any other element.

(c) The element has a direct influence on the organism and is involved in the metabolism of the organism.

The deficiency of the element is observed by abnormal or stunted growth when the element is present in inadequate concentrations in the nutrient intake while serious deficiencies can lead to growth or reproductive failure and even death.

Deficiency disorders can usually be corrected by adding the deficient element to the food supply but this is not invariably so, since the feeding of the appropriate levels of cobalt or its salts does not rectify vitamin B_{12} (cyanocobalamin) deficiency, possibly because this substance is complexed or chelated.

Toxicity can result from too high a concentration of an element and may give rise to abnormal growth, disease or even death. All elements, even essential ones, are toxic at high concentrations but the optimum range of concentrations of the essential element may be narrow as with copper or broad as with calcium or potassium.

Toxicity depends on species and may be modified by the components in the diet supplied. It must be emphasised that individuals are variable in their biological response and while this may occur in a single individual, the variation is greater within the species. Since, for example, different mammals have different responses, any comparison should be made on a steady parameter, which is frequently taken as the dose per unit of body weight and often expressed as milligrams per kilogram of body weight.

There is a paucity of information concerning the deficiencies of a particular element in a diet. Often this occurs because the foodstuffs have never been investigated for the element and hence there may well be a lack of information about the toxicity of that same element in larger quantities in the diet.

So-called "normal" diets may be deficient in some essential elements such as zinc, iron and chromium while relatively large amounts of the so-called poisonous elements such as arsenic and mercury are needed to produce toxicity or death when compared with the amounts present in a diet. Thus for some elements there is a low safety margin between the concentrations normally present and those known to be toxic, e.g., cadmium, lead and fluorine.

As the absorption across the gut wall is poor and variable, toxicity by oral administration is higher than by intravenous injection. This, of course, is true of other substances as well as elements.

Table I shows the effects which deficiencies and excesses of some elements will have upon mammals. In general one refers to man but the effects of excess fluoride on cattle are well known and have been too easily seen in some areas due to atmospheric pollution. Deficiencies of iodine, productive of goitre, or due to its locality—Derbyshire Neck—led to the addition of standardised quantities of potassium or sodium iodide to salt; this was covered by a Code of Practice.[1]

The addition of fluoride to water in order to reduce the incidence of dental caries is highly controversial and fortunately has not reached the Statute Book as opinion is very divided and ill effects of the element may easily be obtained with a slight increase of dose.

Lead is one element which does not occur naturally in the mammalian organism, hence its absence can only be beneficial. It is readily stored, however, and may replace calcium in the composition of bone material while continued intake, even in extremely small quantities, causes deterioration of the brain as well as other organs.

Table I: Effect of Deficiencies and Excesses of Some Elements upon Mammals

Element	Deficiency	Excess
Arsenic	Enlarged spleen, poor growth rate	Stomach pain, goitre, convulsions
Cobalt	Anaemia	Polycythemia, heart failure
Chromium	Corneal opacity, poor glucose metabolism	Lung cancer by inhalation
Copper	Anaemia, hair kinky or depigmented	Jaundice
Fluorine	Poor bones and teeth	Bone sclerosis and mottled teeth
Iron	Anaemia	Siderosis and Haemochromatosis
Iodine	Hypothyroidism Goitre	Hyperthyroidism
Lead	None	Brain damage, neuritis, kidney cancer
Zinc	Dermatitis, dwarfism, immature gonads	Anaemia

Table II shows the same elements as before but now expressed in terms of milligrams per day. The intake from a diet which is deficient in the element is shown together with the normal range of the element and finally the toxic quantity of the element.

Table II: Doses of Some Elements in Human Diets, mg/day

Element	Deficient Diet	Normal Range	Toxic Quantity
Arsenic	0.07	0.04-1.4	5-50
Cobalt	0.0002	0.005-1.8	500
Chromium	0.005	0.01-1.2	200
Copper	0.3	0.5-6	–
Fluorine	–	0.3-5	20
Iron	6	6-40	200
Iodine	0.015	0.1-0.2	2
Lead	–	0.06-0.5	1
Zinc	5	5-40	150-600

This toxic quantity is not necessarily that quantity which produces death, but is any intermediate quantity which interferes with the normal well-being of the individual. Thus, referring to lead, there can be no deficiencies caused by its absence from the diet. However, continued consumption of food contaminated with lead, or indeed exposure to other sources of lead contamination of the environment will speedily lead to some impairment of health.

Various reports have been stated that zinc deficiencies exist in both the U.K. and the U.S.A.; indeed the deficiencies are endemic. A deficiency of zinc also produce stress and tension in the individual. Zinc deficiency may hence be one reason for the generally harassed behaviour of so many civilised people in recent years.

Referring again to Table I, it shows that chromium deficiency is associated with a poor glucose metabolism. This may be corrected by the addition of 500 micrograms of chromium per day which is a very small quantity. This is 0.5 milligram and considering Table II, the quantity is within the normal daily dietary range but is only about 1/400th the toxic quantity.

Table III shows the residence times of some elements in the body. This is the rate at which the element is used by the body and is replaced from dietary and other sources, compared with the amount of the normally, naturally occurring element in the body. The estimates are necessarily only approximate as the factors involved in such a calculation are incompletely known. However, it will be seen that one may expect to have over four years supply of copper and zinc in the body. This highlights the seriousness of deficiencies of such elements, since replacing the natural store cannot be done quickly and is a long and tedious process. One sees this with the treatment of anaemia.

Table III: Residence of Some Elements in the Human Body

Element	Residence Time in Days
Cobalt	100-200
Arsenic	250-400
Copper	800-1,600
Zinc	over 1,600

Naturally there exists an enormous body of information on trace elements and more detailed information may be obtained from *Trace Elements in Human and Animal Nutrition* by E.J. Underwood.[2] Another book of interest is *Soil, Grass and Cancer* by Andre Voisin.[3] This French veterinarian links the health of animals and man to the mineral balance of the soil. The book is rather old (1959) and has not, to my knowledge, been updated. Nevertheless it contains many truisms.

The *Tables of Composition of Foods* published by H.M.S.O.[4] include some trace elements. Perusal of the book shows that particularly rich sources of some of the elements are crustacea, molluscs, spinach and meat (particularly offal), soya and especially defatted soya products.

It must not be forgotten that molluscs and crustaceans concentrate metals and there are some reports on the presence of a strong metallic taste when they are ingested. This exists because these creatures have been filtering off, or living in a medium heavily charged with effluents—even if adequately diluted—which contain metals. This possibly explains the very wide variations reported in the literature for concentrations of metals found in some fish. It will be remembered, that a mussel may filter over 20 litres, i.e., nearly 5 gallons, of water per day through its gills.

EFFECT OF PHYTIC ACID

Cereals and nuts contain a substance known as phytic acid which is a compound of a hexahydric alcohol (inosital) with six molecules of phosphoric acid. As most of this substance occurs in the bran and germ of cereals and these (bran and germ) are removed during the milling process, then normal flours are low in phytic acid. Wholemeal and similarly milled flours are richer in this substance. The drawback to the use of flour containing phytic acid is that it seriously interferes with the absorption of dietary calcium and iron even to the extent of inactivating more calcium than could be taken in from the cereal and acting as a potential inactivator to valuable calcium and iron in the remainder of the diet.[5] This was one of the reasons for "fortification" of white flour during the 1939-45 War. This is still practised and it ensures the adequacy of available calcium and iron in our present day diet.

Oatmeal has a higher phytic acid content than wheatflour and it could be a reason why scholars returning to some of the northern-most Universities in former times took sacks of oatmeal and dried or salted herring. The latter dietary item may well have been to improve the calcium balance of the diet as well as redressing lack of protein.

When cereals are soaked, as in the production of porridge by traditional methods, an enzyme called phytase has the chance to work on and split the phytic acid molecule and render it inactive. The present vogue for "quick" or "instant" oatmeal, etc., with a very short period of soaking may well increase the phytate content actually consumed. Muesli may have a high phytate content hence with advantage could be replaced by alternative forms of cereal.

EFFECTS OF CYANOGENETIC GLUCOSIDES

Beans, a favourite and traditional food, may seem to be unlikely items to cause ill health, yet they are alleged to have caused severe heart attacks in some people. Beyond rather vague reports, no effort appears to have been made to investigate this phenomenon. An additional risk, however, with some beans is the occurrence of cyanogenetic glucosides which may also occur in other seeds and plants used in human and animal nutrition. The glucosides tend to disappear with continued cultivation of the species and of course, should disappear with cooking.[6] In the dried material, as sold, the glucoside and the enzyme which cause the splitting and production of hydrocyanic acid are not in contact, hence no hydrocyanic acid production occurs.

If consumed dry, the body temperature is one of the most favourable for enzyme action and mastication brings the two substances together. Usually temperatures over 60°C will destroy the enzyme, hence under normal conditions, cooking destroys the glucoside and the cyanide portion disappears harmlessly.

Other toxic factors appear to exist in beans and numerous reports have been made on the use of red kidney beans either uncooked as in bean salads or Mexican salad, or added late during the cooking of a stew such as chili con carne.[6b,c,d] In other words, the stew put on in the morning may be thoroughly cooked but the beans added by a shopper returning late from work may be insufficiently cooked and be toxic. Had this ingredient received the same length of cooking as the others it would have been satisfactory.

The following factors, known to be destroyed by prolonged cooking have been identified in red beans.[6e]

(a) A goitrogen.

(b) A trypsin inhibitor–this stimulates the overproduction of digestive enzymes by the pancreas.

(c) Haemaglutinins which probably impair absorption of digestive products.

The existence of this haemaglutinin has been known for some time and was a cause for alarm in the early 1970's when the seeds of *Abrus precatorius* were being widely imported in the form of necklaces, brought back by tourists from North Africa and the Caribbean area. The seeds were better known as Jequirity beans and were pierced to form the necklace. The bean thus became potentially dangerous as it is much safer if the seed coat is intact. Boiling would have destroyed the toxic nature of the seed but drying does not.

The haemaglutinin was classified a considerable time ago as a toxalbumin and the properties of this substance resemble crotin from crotin seeds and ricin from castor seeds, but although the properties are similar, the substances are not identical.

It is quite possible for the beans to pass through the intestinal tract without harm, providing the mucosa are intact but the slightest laceration enables the toxic principles to be absorbed with frequently fatal results. Advantage was taken of the agglutinating property of the toxalbumins when Markov was shot in this country and a compatriot of his in France using a pellet probably coated with an extract from such seeds. Both of these events occurred since 1976.

Mention has already been made of the cyanogenetic glucosides and it must be pointed out that many green vegetables, especially members of the Brassica family such as cabbage, sprouts, etc., may contain up to 0.1% of these substances. Usually they are consumed after cooking when the glucoside has been destroyed, but "party dips" using cauliflower heads and of course cole slaw with uncooked cabbage may contain un-changed glucoside.

Even cooked cabbage is not necessarily free from this as the following example demonstrates. An investigation was being made in blood circulatory rate, and recovery tests in excreta were being performed, when one patient produced a result several times greater than the quantity of cyanide injected; this was correlated with tachycardia. Enquiry elicited the information that the patient had consumed a large portion of cabbage before the test. It was subsequently confirmed that large servings of cabbage and related vegetables, especially if undercooked, could produce similar results.[7]

The nature or consumption of these glucosides is not always known with precision. A similar compound does exist, however, in some species of leguminosae especially white cloves, which has a goitrogenic effect due to contained thiocyanate. Narrow stem kale, and even the milk of cows fed on narrow stem kale, contains a sufficient quantity of this factor to have a significant goitrogenic effect upon consumers.[8a,b,c]

THE EFFECTS OF HISTAMINE PRODUCTION

Much more unexpected is the apparent effect on some people of consumption of smoked mackerel. For sometime it has been known that poisonous fish occur even in northern waters, while other species of fish at spawning time may occasionally produce mass poisoning. Within the last three years a number of cases of poisoning have occurred after consumption of mackerel. Similar cases have arisen with bonito, tuna and skipjack all of which are readily available in the United Kingdom either fresh, canned, deep frozen or in prepared dishes. All of these fish belong to the family Scombroidae and this family includes mackerel.

Persons who have suffered from this form of poisoning complain that the fish has a sharp or peppery taste and after consumption, symptoms may occur in a short period, one hour being usual but up to three hours is not unknown. The symptoms are head pains, flushes, dizziness and possibly an itching rash, while less commonly nausea and diarrhoea occur. It has been claimed that death may result in very severe cases.[9]

In Britain the symptoms have been short lived and recovery has occurred in hours rather than days, sometimes without medical intervention.

These fish all contain a heterocyclic amino acid, hisitidine, which by decarboxylation becomes histamine:

$$\text{Histidine} \xrightarrow{-CO_2} \text{Histamine}$$

Histidine: imidazole ring—CH_2CHNH_2 with $COOH$

Histamine: imidazole ring—$CH_2CH_2NH_2$

This reaction is caused by bacteria, especially of the Proteous species and high levels of histamine are often produced before the fish becomes unacceptable. Unacceptability from this cause must not be confused with decomposition which may be occurring at the same time.

The levels of histamine which cause trouble are usually over 25 mg histamine per 100 g fish. It has been suggested that if histamine levels of between 10 and 20 mg per 100 g fish are exceeded then the fish should be rejected as unsuitable. With 100 mg histamine or more per 100 gm fish, susceptible individuals are almost certain to have problems.[10]

Attempts have been made without success to find substances other than histamine which will cause these symptoms. The presence of such other substances has hence been doubted but the search continues.

It is quite likely that the recent increase in this unexpected poisoning is due to the following facts:

(a) Closure to Britain of traditional bottom feeding grounds which has led to an increase in the quantity of mackerel caught and processed.

(b) The sales of hot smoked mackerel have increased, and it may be that a number of processors with inadequate knowledge and possibly lower standards of hygiene have entered the industry.

(c) The organisms causing the change are normally present in the fish; the toxins produced are not destroyed by heat even at canning temperatures. From time of catch to processing the fish should be kept at a temperature below 4°C.

It must not be overlooked that Proteous organisms occur in sewage and sewage effluents and the sea waters around the British coast are increasingly polluted with these waste products. Mackerel are known to be "dirty" feeders so they may initially become contaminated with Proteous in this way.

Another unusual incident involved the reaction by a teacher and some children to sardines. Within a few minutes after eating they were all affected by red blotches on the cheeks and irritation. A further group of children ate the sardines between slices of bread and were not affected. The symptoms disappeared within one to two hours and suggested mild scombroid poisoning. Opened and unopened cans of the sardines were analysed and found to contain 85 mg histamine per 100 g sardine in unopened cans and 83 mg per 100 g fish in the opened can, confirming both the high level of histamine and the probable cause of the poisoning.

Histamine is rapidly absorbed through the mucous membranes of the mouth but when swallowed the histamine is inactivated in the stomach. When eating the sardines in the form of a sandwich, much less fish comes into contact with the mouth and no symptoms develop.[11] It is likely that the fish had undergone a measure of spoilage before they were canned and the temperature of processing was too low to destroy the amine.

CONCLUSIONS

Many other papers and books have been published mentioning the presence of solanine in immature potatoes, ergot in bread, oxalates in sorrel and rhubarb, as well as fungal poisoning due to mistaken identity. The use of absinthe in wines has been largely prohibited or limited in various countries since habitual consumption produces vomiting, vertigo and convulsions.

Of necessity, this has been a very brief review and many subjects have been omitted, but it is hoped that enough has been written to stimulate interest into what is frequently an almost overlooked or forgotten subject. The wholesomeness of food is nowadays taken for granted and, while the food may conform to various criteria when purchased, this is not always a sufficient guarantee unless it is subsequently thoroughly cooked.

REFERENCES

(1)   Code of Practice of the Local Authorities Joint Advisory Committee on Food Standards No. 11 (H.M.S.O., London, 1950).
(2)   E.J. Underwood, *Trace Elements in Human and Animal Nutrition* (Academic Press, London, 1977).
(3)   A. Voisin, *Soil, Grass and Cancer* (Crosby Lockwood, London, 1959).
(4)   McCance and Widdowson's the Composition of Foods, Ed. A.A. Paul and D.A.T. Southgate, 4th Ed. (H.M.S.O., London, 1978).
(5)   D.W. Kent-Jones and A.J. Amos, *Modern Cereal Chemistry* 6th Ed. (Free Trade Press, London, 1967).
(6a) C.R. Gunn, *Garden J.* 88 (Jan/Feb. 1969).
(6b) Anon, *Brit Med. J.* 2, 1268 (1976).
(6c) D. Roberts, *Environmental Health* 85, 216 (1977).
(6d) R.G. Fidoe, *idem* 87, 47 (1979).
      M.S. Shafi, *idem* 87, 47 (1979).
(6e) J. Smart, *Tropical Pulses* (Tropical Agriculture Series) (Longmans, London, 1976).
(7)   G.V. James, *Analyst*, 64, 500 (1939).
(8a) D.S. Flux, G.W. Butler and J.M. Johnson, *New Zealand J. of Sci & Tech.* 38 (A), 88 (1956).
(8b) A. Shand, *Brit. Veterinary Assoc. Public* No. 23, 58 91952).
(8c) F.W. Clements and J.W. Wishart, *Metabolism* 5, 623 (1956).
(9)   S.H. Arnold and W.D. Brown, Histamine Toxicity from Fish Products in *Advances in Food Research* (Academic Press 24, 114-154, 1978).
(10) C. Murray, Torry Research Station, Aberdeen Private Communication (1980).
(11) R.A. Dalley, *The Official Analyst* 1, 10 (1981).

Index

(Authors' names are only given if they appear in the text and not just in the list of references at the end of chapters.)